Children, Adolescents, and the Media

Guest Editor

VICTOR C. STRASBURGER, MD

PEDIATRIC CLINICS
OF NORTH AMERICA

www.pediatric.theclinics.com

June 2012 • Volume 59 • Number 3

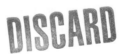
SAUNDERS an imprint of ELSEVIER, Inc.

W.B. SAUNDERS COMPANY
A Division of Elsevier Inc.

1600 John F. Kennedy Boulevard • Suite 1800 • Philadelphia, Pennsylvania 19103-2899

http://www.theclinics.com

THE PEDIATRIC CLINICS OF NORTH AMERICA Volume 59, Number 3
June 2012 ISSN 0031-3955, ISBN-13: 978-1-4557-4681-1

Editor: Kerry Holland
Developmental Editor: Donald Mumford

Photocopying
Single photocopies of single articles may be made for personal use as allowed by national copyright laws. Permission of the Publisher and payment of a fee is required for all other photocopying, including multiple or systematic copying, copying for advertising or promotional purposes, resale, and all forms of document delivery. Special rates are available for educational institutions that wish to make photocopies for non-profit educational classroom use. For information on how to seek permission visit www.elsevier.com/permissions or call: (+44) 1865 843830 (UK)/(+1) 215 239 3804 (USA).

Derivative Works
Subscribers may reproduce tables of contents or prepare lists of articles including abstracts for internal circulation within their institutions. Permission of the Publisher is required for resale or distribution outside the institution. Permission of the Publisher is required for all other derivative works, including compilations and translations (please consult www.elsevier.com/permissions).

Electronic Storage or Usage
Permission of the Publisher is required to store or use electronically any material contained in this journal, including any article or part of an article (please consult www.elsevier.com/permissions). Except as outlined above, no part of this publication may be reproduced, stored in a retrieval system or transmitted in any form or by any means, electronic, mechanical, photocopying, recording or otherwise, without prior written permission of the Publisher.

Notice
No responsibility is assumed by the Publisher for any injury and/or damage to persons or property as a matter of products liability, negligence or otherwise, or from any use or operation of any methods, products, instructions or ideas contained in the material herein. Because of rapid advances in the medical sciences, in particular, independent verification of diagnoses and drug dosages should be made.

Although all advertising material is expected to conform to ethical (medical) standards, inclusion in this publication does not constitute a guarantee or endorsement of the quality or value of such product or of the claims made of it by its manufacturer.

The Pediatric Clinics of North America (ISSN 0031-3955) is published bimonthly by Elsevier Inc., 360 Park Avenue South, New York, NY 10010-1710. Months of issue are February, April, June, August, October, and December. Periodicals postage paid at New York, NY and additional mailing offices. Subscription prices are $191.00 per year (US individuals), $444.00 per year (US institutions), $259.00 per year (Canadian individuals), $591.00 per year (Canadian institutions), $308.00 per year (international individuals), $591.00 per year (international institutions), $93.00 per year (US students and residents), and $159.00 per year (international and Canadian residents and students). To receive students/resident rare, orders must be accompanied by name of affiliated institution, date of term, and the signature of program/residency coordinator on institution letterhead. Orders will be billed at individual rate until proof of status is received. Foreign air speed delivery is included in all *Clinics* subscription prices. All prices are subject to change without notice. **POSTMASTER:** Send address changes to *The Pediatric Clinics of North America*, Elsevier Health Sciences Division, Subscription Customer Service, 3251 Riverport Lane, Maryland Heights, MO 63043. **Customer Service: 1-800-654-2452 (US and Canada). From outside of the US and Canada: 1-314-447-8871. Fax: 1-314-447-8029. For print support, E-mail: JournalsCustomerService-usa@elsevier.com. For online support, E-mail: JournalsOnlineSupport-usa@elsevier.com.**

Reprints. For copies of 100 or more, of articles in this publication, please contact the Commercial Reprints Department, Elsevier Inc., 360 Park Avenue South, New York, NY 10010-1710. Tel.: 212-633-3812; Fax: 212-462-1935; E-mail: reprints@elsevier.com.

The Pediatric Clinics of North America is also published in Spanish by McGraw-Hill Inter-americana Editores S.A., Mexico City, Mexico; in Portuguese by Riechmann and Affonso Editores, Rua Comandante Coelho 1085, CEP 21250, Rio de Janeiro, Brazil; and in Greek by Althayia SA, Athens, Greece.

The Pediatric Clinics of North America is covered in *MEDLINE/PubMed (Index Medicus), Excerpta Medica, Current Contents, Current Contents/Clinical Medicine, Science Citation Index, ASCA, ISI/BIOMED,* and *BIOSIS.*

Printed in the United States of America.

GOAL STATEMENT

The goal of the *Pediatric Clinics of North America* is to keep practicing physicians and residents up to date with current clinical practice in pediatrics by providing timely articles reviewing the state-of-the-art in patient care.

ACCREDITATION

The *Pediatric Clinics of North America* is planned and implemented in accordance with the Essential Areas and Policies of the Accreditation Council for Continuing Medical Education (ACCME) through the joint sponsorship of the University Of Virginia School Of Medicine and Elsevier. The University Of Virginia School of Medicine is accredited by the ACCME to provide continuing medical education for physicians.

The University of Virginia School of Medicine designates this enduring material activity for a maximum of 15 *AMA PRA Category 1 Credit*(s)™ for each issue, 90 credits per year. Physicians should only claim credit commensurate with the extent of their participation in the activity.

The American Medical Association has determined that physicians not licensed in the US who participate in this CME enduring material activity are eligible for a maximum of 15 *AMA PRA Category 1 Credit*(s)™ for each issue, 90 credits per year.

Credit can be earned by reading the text material, taking the CME examination online at http://www.theclinics.com/home/cme, and completing the evaluation. After taking the test, you will be required to review any and all incorrect answers. Following completion of the test and evaluation, your credit will be awarded and you may print your certificate.

FACULTY DISCLOSURE/CONFLICT OF INTEREST

The University of Virginia School of Medicine, as an ACCME accredited provider, endorses and strives to comply with the Accreditation Council for Continuing Medical Education (ACCME) Standards of Commercial Support, Commonwealth of Virginia statutes, University of Virginia policies and procedures, and associated federal and private regulations and guidelines on the need for disclosure and monitoring of proprietary and financial interests that may affect the scientific integrity and balance of content delivered in continuing medical education activities under our auspices.

The University of Virginia School of Medicine requires that all CME activities accredited through this institution be developed independently and be scientifically rigorous, balanced and objective in the presentation/discussion of its content, theories and practices.

All authors/editors participating in an accredited CME activity are expected to disclose to the readers relevant financial relationships with commercial entities occurring within the past 12 months (such as grants or research support, employee, consultant, stock holder, member of speakers bureau, etc.). The University of Virginia School of Medicine will employ appropriate mechanisms to resolve potential conflicts of interest to maintain the standards of fair and balanced education to the reader. Questions about specific strategies can be directed to the Office of Continuing Medical Education, University of Virginia School of Medicine, Charlottesville, Virginia.

The faculty and staff of the University of Virginia Office of Continuing Medical Education have no financial affiliations to disclose.

The authors/editors listed below have identified no financial or professional relationships for themselves or their spouse/partner:
Craig A. Anderson, PhD; Carson A. Benowitz-Fredericks, BA; Dina L.G. Borzekowski, EdD; Jeff Chester, MSW; Ed Donnerstein, PhD; Lori Dorfman, DrPH; Kaylor Garcia, BA; Douglas A. Gentile, PhD; Sonya A. Grier, MBA, PhD; Melanie Hingle, PhD, MPH, RD; Marjorie J. Hogan, MD; Kerry Holland, (Acquisitions Editor); Jennifer Kolb, MD; Amy B. Jordan, PhD; Dale Kunkel, PhD; Alexis R. Lauricella, PhD; Meredith Massey, EdM; Cathy McCarthy, MPH; Katelyn A. McDonald, ; Kathryn C. Montgomery, PhD; Megan A. Moreno, MD, MSEd, MPH; Sara Prot, MA; Karen Rheuban, MD (Test Author); Brintha Vasagar, MD, MPH; and Ellen A. Wartella, PhD.

The authors/editors listed below identified the following professional or financial affiliations for themselves or their spouse/partner:
Gwenn SchurginO'Keeffe, MD is employed by Pull Ups, Cutter Insect Repellent, Barilla Nutrition, MedHealth Systems, ONDCP Social Media Technical Panel, and the Harvard Pilgrim LinkedIn Group Expert.
Walter D. Rosenfeld, MD is a consultant for Pfizer, Inc.
Victor C. Strasburger, MD (Guest Editor) is on the Speakers' Bureau for Merck.

Disclosure of Discussion of Non-FDA Approved Uses for Pharmaceutical Products and/or Medical Devices

The University of Virginia School of Medicine, as an ACCME provider, requires that all faculty presenters identify and disclose any off-label uses for pharmaceutical and medical device products. The University of Virginia School of Medicine recommends that each physician fully review all the available data on new products or procedures prior to clinical use.

TO ENROLL

To enroll in the Pediatric Clinics of North America Continuing Medical Education program, call customer service at 1-800-654-2452 or visit us online at www.theclinics.com/home/cme. The CME program is available to subscribers for an additional fee of $223.00.

Contributors

GUEST EDITOR

VICTOR C. STRASBURGER, MD
Professor of Pediatrics, Professor of Family & Community Medicine, Chief, Department of Pediatrics, Division of Adolescent Medicine, University of New Mexico School of Medicine, Albuquerque, New Mexico

AUTHORS

CRAIG A. ANDERSON, PhD
Distinguished Professor, Department of Psychology, Iowa State University, Ames, Iowa

CARSON A. BENOWITZ-FREDERICKS, BA
Department of Health, Behavior and Society, Johns Hopkins Bloomberg School of Public Health, Baltimore, Maryland

DINA L.G. BORZEKOWSKI, EdD
Associate Professor, Department of Health, Behavior and Society, Johns Hopkins Bloomberg School of Public Health, Baltimore, Maryland

JEFF CHESTER, MSW
Executive Director, Center for Digital Democracy, Washington, DC

ED DONNERSTEIN, PhD
Department of Communication, University of Arizona, Tucson, Arizona

LORI DORFMAN, DrPH
Director, Berkeley Media Studies Group, Berkeley, California

KAYLOR GARCIA, BA
Department of Health, Behavior and Society, Johns Hopkins Bloomberg School of Public Health, Baltimore, Maryland

DOUGLAS A. GENTILE, PhD
Associate Professor, Department of Psychology, Iowa State University, Ames, Iowa

SONYA A. GRIER, MBA, PhD
Associate Professor, Department of Marketing, Kogod School of Business, American University, Washington, DC

MELANIE HINGLE, PhD, MPH, RD
Assistant Research Professor, Department of Nutritional Sciences, University of Arizona, Tucson, Arizona

MARJORIE J. HOGAN, MD
Department of Pediatrics, Hennepin County Medical Center; Associate Professor of Pediatrics, University of Minnesota, Minneapolis, Minnesota

AMY B. JORDAN, PhD
Media and Developing Child Sector, Annenberg Public Policy Center, University of Pennsylvania, Philadelphia, Pennsylvania

JENNIFER KOLB, MD
Pediatric Resident, Department of Pediatrics, University of Wisconsin–Madison, Madison, Wisconsin

DALE KUNKEL, PhD
Professor, Department of Communication, University of Arizona, Tucson, Arizona

ALEXIS R. LAURICELLA, PhD
Postdoctoral Fellow, Northwestern University, Evanston, Illinois

MEREDITH MASSEY, EdM
Department of Health, Behavior and Society, Johns Hopkins Bloomberg School of Public Health, Baltimore, Maryland

CATHY MCCARTHY, MPH
Morristown Medical Center, Atlantic Health System, Morristown, New Jersey

KATELYN A. MCDONALD
Student, Department of Psychology, Iowa State University, Ames, Iowa

KATHRYN C. MONTGOMERY, PhD
Professor, School of Communication, American University, Washington, DC

MEGAN A. MORENO, MD, MSEd, MPH
Assistant Professor, Department of Pediatrics, University of Wisconsin–Madison, Madison, Wisconsin

GWENN SCHURGIN O'KEEFFE, MD, FAAP
CEO and Editor in Chief, Pediatrics Now, Wayland, Massachusetts

SARA PROT, MA
Doctoral Student, Department of Psychology, Iowa State University, Ames, Iowa

WALTER D. ROSENFELD, MD
Goryeb Children's Hospital, Atlantic Health System, Morristown, New Jersey

VICTOR C. STRASBURGER, MD
Professor of Pediatrics, Professor of Family & Community Medicine, Chief, Department of Pediatrics, Division of Adolescent Medicine, University of New Mexico School of Medicine, Albuquerque, New Mexico

BRINTHA VASAGAR, MD, MPH
Department of Health, Behavior and Society, Johns Hopkins Bloomberg School of Public Health, Baltimore, Maryland

ELLEN A. WARTELLA, PhD
Al-Thani Professor of Communication, Professor of Psychology; Professor of Human Development and Social Policy; Director, Center on Media and Human Development, Northwestern University, Evanston, Illinois

Contents

The media can be a powerful teacher of children and adolescents and have a profound impact on their health. The media are not the leading cause of *any* major health problem in the United States, but they *do* contribute to a variety of pediatric and adolescent health problems. Given that children and teens spend >7 hours a day with media, one would think that adult society would recognize its impact on young people's attitudes and behaviors. Too little has been done to protect children and adolescents from harmful media effects and to maximize the powerfully prosocial aspects of modern media.

Pediatricians care for children's growth and development from the time they are born until they become adults. In addition, pediatricians must be vigilant for external influences. Technology influences children of all ages. Seventy-five percent of teenagers own cell phones, with 25% using them for social media. Technology can lead to an increase in skills and social benefits but there is also the potential for harm such as sexting, cyberbullying, privacy issues, and Internet addiction, all of which can affect health. Pediatricians must become well versed in the new media to provide media-oriented anticipatory guidance and advice on media-related issues.

Social networking sites are popular among and consistently used by adolescents. These sites present benefits as well as risks to adolescent health. Recently, pediatric providers have also considered the benefits and risks of using social networking sites in their own practices.

Should babies be watching television and DVDs? This is a reasonable question to ask but a difficult one to answer. This article reviews the theories and related research to examine what is known about infant media use. The review provides evidence both for and against each theory. The importance of infants learning how to watch and learn from screen media presentations is indicated and the new world of media to which babies are exposed is discussed.

This article assesses the role played by media in contributing to the current epidemic of childhood obesity. Electronic media use, often referred to as screen time, is significantly correlated with child adiposity. Although the causal mechanism that accounts for this relationship is unclear, it is well established that reducing screen time improves weight status. Media advertising for unhealthy foods contributes to obesity by influencing children's food preferences, requests, and diet. Industry efforts have failed to improve the nutritional quality of foods marketed on television to children, leading public health advocates to recommend government restrictions on child-targeted advertisements for unhealthy foods.

Historically and currently, media messages around body shape and size emphasize the importance of being below-average weight for women and hypermuscular for men. The media messages around physical appearance are not realistic for most and lead to body dissatisfaction for most adolescents. Interventions designed to mitigate the influence of negative media messages on adolescents' body image are presented; however, most have shown limited success.

Most American schools are 50 years behind in incorporating new technology into the classroom and using media wisely. Some experts estimate that 65% of today's grade-school students may end up doing jobs that have not even been invented yet. Abundant evidence now exists that children and teens learn preferentially from the media, yet the media are often frowned on as too distracting for students or too distant from the basic 3 Rs. American schools are failing in their fundamental responsibility to students. Educators need to learn how to use media and new technology wisely.

The Internet, in contrast to in-person interactions with health providers, allows anonymous and nonpunitive ease of access. Adolescents have long sought honest, direct answers to important but embarrassing questions about health; emerging technologies provide a venue to obtain relevant information without geographic, time, financial, and personal barriers. This article is a case study of TeenHealthFX.com. Those interested in how youth access online health information can learn of the positive and negative aspects of delivering messages through the Internet. This article discusses the process involved in creating and maintaining TeenHealthFX and the challenges of providing online health information to adolescents via new technology.

Children, Adolescents, and the Media

PEDIATRIC CLINICS
OF NORTH AMERICA

DOWNLOAD
Free App!

Review Articles
THE CLINICS

NOW AVAILABLE FOR YOUR iPhone and iPad

Preface

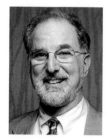

Victor C. Strasburger, MD
Guest Editor

It is a complete mystery to me why some people don't "get it" — the media represent one of the most powerful forces shaping young people's lives today. Potentially, the media can have an effect on virtually *every* concern that parents and pediatricians have about children and adolescents — sex, drugs, aggressive behavior, school performance, obesity, eating disorders, even sleep. And when young people are now spending 7-11 hours a day with media, it seems like a no-brainer. So why don't some people understand this?

I hope this issue of *Pediatric Clinics* will go a long way in convincing the nay-sayers that media are not only important, they are now *crucial* in young people's lives. And that media can be a force for good or not-so-good. Yo — Hollywood and Madison Avenue — we do not hate you. We just wish you would understand that with the billions of dollars you make every year, you have a public health responsibility as well. As we adolescent medicine specialists always counsel parents *never* to say to their teenagers: we wish you would do better! American media are absolutely *amazing* sometimes in a good and positive way (I'll just mention TV shows like *Sesame Street*, *The Wire*, *Modern Family*, *Glee*, and *Nature* and a few recent movies like *March of the Penguins*, *Toy Story*, *Hugo*, *War Horse*, *The King's Speech*, and *Bully*).

I want to thank Kerry Holland at Elsevier for her support and encouragement for doing this issue and all of the authors — who are some of the finest minds in the field of American media — for contributing their expertise.

Victor C. Strasburger, MD
Department of Pediatrics
Division of Adolescent Medicine
University of New Mexico School of Medicine
MSC10 5590, 1 University of New Mexico
Albuquerque, NM 87131, USA

E-mail address:
VStrasburger@salud.unm.edu

doi:10.1016/j.pcl.2012.03.028
pediatric.theclinics.com

Children, Adolescents, and the Media: Health Effects

Victor C. Strasburger, MD[a],*, Amy B. Jordan, PhD[b],
Ed Donnerstein, PhD[c]

KEYWORDS

• Media • TV • New technology • Internet • Cyberbullying • Sexting • Media literacy

KEY POINTS

- Young people now spend 7 to 11 hours per day with a variety of different media—more time than they spend in school or sleeping.
- Research has shown that children and teenagers learn from the media, and their behavior can be influenced by media.
- Media can have significant effects on health: eg, obesity, aggressive behavior, substance use, early sexual activity, eating disorders.
- Media can be powerfully prosocial at times.
- Parents, clinicians, and schools need to adapt to the world of new technology and understand the influence that media can have on young people.

> True, media violence is not likely to turn an otherwise fine child into a violent criminal. But, just as every cigarette one smokes increases a little bit the likelihood of a lung tumor someday, every violent show one watches increases just a little bit the likelihood of behaving more aggressively in some situation.
> —Psychologists Brad Bushman and L. Rowell Huesmann[1(p248)]

> "Something's in the air, and I wouldn't call it love. Like never before, our kids are being bombarded by images of oversexed, underdressed celebrities who can't seem to step out of a car without displaying their well-waxed private parts to photographers."
> —Lead article, Newsweek, February 12, 2007[2]

> One erect penis on a US screen is more incendiary than a thousand guns.
> —Newsweek critic David Ansen[3(p66)]

[a] Department of Pediatrics, Division of Adolescent Medicine, University of New Mexico School of Medicine, MSC10 5590, 1 University of New Mexico, Albuquerque, NM 87131, USA; [b] Media and Developing Child Sector, Annenberg Public Policy Center, University of Pennsylvania, 202 South 36th Street, Philadelphia, PA 19104-6220, USA; [c] Department of Communication, University of Arizona, 1103 East University Boulevard, PO Box 210025, Tucson, AZ 85721, USA
* Corresponding author.
E-mail address: VStrasburger@salud.unm.edu

Pediatr Clin N Am 59 (2012) 533–587
doi:10.1016/j.pcl.2012.03.025
0031-3955/12/$ – see front matter © 2012 Elsevier Inc. All rights reserved.

A cigarette in the hands of a Hollywood star onscreen is a gun aimed at a 12- or 14-year-old.

—Screenwriter Joe Eszterhas[4]

Research shows that virtually all women are ashamed of their bodies. It used to be adult women, teenage girls, who were ashamed, but now you see the shame down to very young girls—10, 11 years old. Society's standard of beauty is an image that is literally just short of starvation for most women.

—Best-selling author Mary Pipher[5]

[My doctor's] only gone to one medical school, but if you go online, you can get advice from all over the world.

—Teenager quoted in TECHsex USA, 2011[6(p17)]

We are doing our youth a disservice if we believe that we can protect them from the world by limiting their access to public life. They must enter that arena, make mistakes, and learn from them. Our role as adults is not to be their policemen, but to be their guide.

—danah boyd, 2007[7]

Media represent one of the most powerful and underappreciated influences on child and adolescent development and health. More than 50 years of media research and thousands of media effects studies attest to the potential power of the media to influence virtually every concern that parents and clinicians have about young people: aggressive behavior, sex, drugs, obesity, eating disorders, school performance, suicide, and depression.[8] Although the media cannot be accused of being the leading cause of any of these health problems, they can make a substantial contribution. Yet media can also be powerfully beneficial in the lives of children and adolescents. Not only can they teach young children numbers and letters and increase school readiness (eg, *Sesame Street*),[9] the media can also teach more abstract concepts like empathy, acceptance of diversity, and respect for the elderly.[10,11] Clearly, much more research is needed,[12] but clinicians, parents, school administrators, and government officials all need to be aware of the research on the effects of modern media and act accordingly (**Fig. 1**).

"OLD" VERSUS "NEW" MEDIA

According to a recent report, media represent the leading leisure-time activity for both children and adolescents (**Fig. 2**).[13] Young people spend more than 7 hours a day with a variety of different media, but despite the onslaught of new media "gadgets"

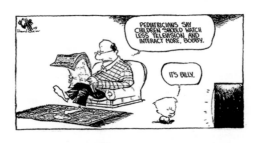

Fig. 1. (Copyright © Patrick O'Connor/*The Kent-Ravenna*, Ohio Record Courier. Used with permission.)

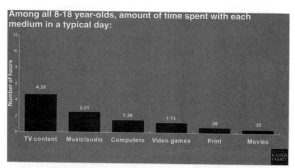

Fig. 2. Children spend >7 hours a day with a variety of different media. (*Reproduced with permission from* Kaiser Family Foundation.)

(**Fig. 3**),[14] TV remains the predominant medium, even for teenagers (**Fig. 4**). Presence of a bedroom TV increases the average number of hours of media use to more than 11 hours per day (**Fig. 5**)[13,15] and increases the risk of obesity by 31%,[16] doubles the risk of smoking,[17] diminishes sleep,[18] and lessens participation in hobbies and reading.[8] It also lessens the ability of parents to monitor their children's viewing habits (**Fig. 6**).[19] Television viewing is now at an all-time high in the United States.[20] Black and Hispanic children spend 5 to 6 hours per day watching TV, compared with 3.5 hours for white youth.[13,21] What has changed is that TV is not necessarily viewed on the television set in the den anymore; increasingly, teens are downloading shows to their computers, their iPhones, their iPads, and their cell phones. About 60% of young people's TV viewing consists of live TV on a TV set, but the other 40% is now either time-shifted or watched online, on mobile devices, or DVDs.[13] Less than 30% say that there are parental rules about how much time they can spend watching TV.[13]

But "new" technology has become increasingly important as well. Six years ago, nearly one-third of 8- to 18-year-olds surveyed had Internet access or a computer in their bedroom.[19] The increasing availability of laptop computers in homes, as well as wireless Internet access, means that children today can go online anywhere, at

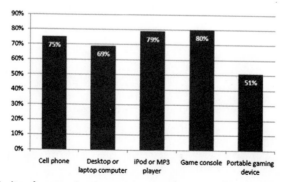

Fig. 3. The popularity of new technology with teenagers. (*From* Lenhart A, Ling R, Campbell S, et al. Teens and Mobile Phones. Pew Internet & American Life Project, April 20, 2010. Available at: http://pewinternet.org/~/media//Files/Reports/2010/PIP-Teens-and-Mobile-2010-with-topline.pdf.)

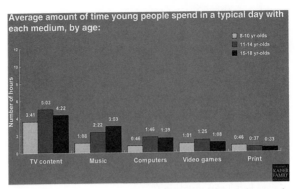

Fig. 4. Even for teenagers, TV remains the predominant medium. (*Reproduced with permission from* Kaiser Family Foundation.)

any time. Half of 8- to 18-year-olds say that they have a video game player in their room.[13] Common Sense Media conducted a survey with a nationally representative sample of children ages 0 to 8. Their findings drive home the fact that media use begins early, and that media technology is widely available in homes with very young children.[22]

- More than a third (39%) of children 8 and younger live in homes where the television is left on all or most of the time, whether or not anyone is watching it.
- Of children 8 and younger, 42% have a TV in their bedroom, and most live in a home with a computer (72%) and high-speed Internet (68%).
- More than half (52%) of homes with young children own a smartphone, a video iPod, an iPad, or a similar tablet device. About 1 in 4 parents of 0- to 8-year-olds say they have downloaded an "app" for their children (although most parents of children this age admit that they do not know what an "app" is).

Both the Nielsen Company and the Pew Internet & American Life Project have been tracking new media use among adolescents, and their studies highlight the immersive media environment of young people's lives, particularly their social lives[23,24]:

- American 18-year-olds now average nearly 40 hours per week online from their home computers, including 5.5 hours of streaming video.

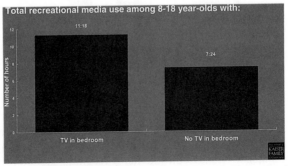

Fig. 5. The presence of a TV in the bedroom increases screen time considerably. (*Reproduced with permission from* Kaiser Family Foundation.)

Media Exposure, by TV Environment and Rules

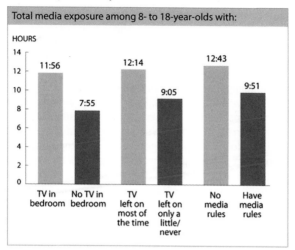

Total media exposure among 8- to 18-year-olds with:

HOURS

- TV in bedroom: 11:56
- No TV in bedroom: 7:55
- TV left on most of the time: 12:14
- TV left on only a little/never: 9:05
- No media rules: 12:43
- Have media rules: 9:51

Fig. 6. Presence of a bedroom TV neutralizes parents' ability to monitor screen time. (*Reproduced with permission from* Kaiser Family Foundation.)

- Nearly all teenagers (93%) now use the Internet. In a 2009 survey, 70% of 12- to 17-year-olds owned a cell phone, and 80% owned an iPod and a game console.
- More than 78% of 12- to 17-year-olds have visited social networks or read blogs.
- Some 75% of 12- to 17-year-olds now own cell phones, up from 45% in 2004. Nearly all teens (88%) are texters.
- Teenagers actually talk less on their phones than any other age group except for seniors. But in the first 3 months of 2011, teens 13 to 17 sent an average of 3364 texts per month. Half of teens send 50 or more text messages per day and one-third send more than 100 per day.
- Teenage boys typically send and receive 30 texts a day; girls 80 texts per day.
- Of 12- to 17-year-olds, 26% say that they have been bullied or harassed via text messages or phone calls. Only 4% say that they have sent a nude or nearly nudge image of themselves to someone else ("sexting"), but 15% say that they have received such a text.
- Half of all cell-phone–owning teens ages 16 to 17 say that they have talked on their phone while driving; one-third say that they have been texting while driving.

Virtually *all* teenagers now have MP3 players, and they often use high-volume settings.[25] Adolescents are notorious multitaskers: nearly 40% of 7th to 12th graders say that they multitask frequently, listening to music (43%), using the computer (40%), or watching TV (39%).[13] Some neuroscientists worry about how efficient multitasking really is and its impact on the developing adolescent brain.[26,27]

Slowly, the changes in media platforms and media use are changing adult society in significant ways as well. For example, the Internet is slowly closing in on TV as Americans' source of national and international news.[28] Many observers feel that the media have a major impact on presidential elections. The average sound bit has decreased from more than 40 seconds in the 1968 election to an average of 7.8 seconds in the 2004 election.[29,30] Other possible behavioral implications of all of this media use are discussed as follows.

HOW DO MEDIA AFFECT CHILDREN AND ADOLESCENTS?

Considerable research attests to the fact that the media can be powerful teachers of young people, shaping their attitudes, beliefs, and behaviors.[8] There are many theories to explain exactly how this might occur, but first the *displacement effect* must be acknowledged: when children and teens spend more than 7 hours a day with media, those are hours that are not spent outside playing, reading a book, or talking with friends. Three of the most appealing theories of media effects are (1) Social Learning Theory, (2) Script or Schema Theory, and (3) "Super-Peer" Theory. According to social learning theory, children and teens learn by observing and imitating attractive role models, precisely what they see on the TV or movie screen, particularly when they see behaviors that are realistic or rewarded.[31] For preteens and teens, "script theory" is extremely relevant, as the media present youth with common "scripts" for how to behave in unfamiliar situations, such as in romantic relationships.[32] Finally, the "super-peer" theory, originally proposed by Strasburger in 1995,[33] states that the media exert inordinate pressure on children and teens to engage in what is depicted as being normative behavior (eg, everyone drinks at a party). The importance of peer pressure on adolescent behavior is universally acknowledged; the media function as a super-peer.[33,34]

Given the abundant research on harmful media effects and the time that young people spend with media, one might think that parents and society in general would be quite cautious and concerned about letting children be exposed to seemingly unending violence, sex, drugs, and commercialism. However, the "third-person effect" seems to mitigate against such concern: teenagers, parents, and adults think that the media affect everyone else except themselves or their children.[35,36] This phenomenon is well-documented in the communications literature.

VIOLENCE AND AGGRESSIVE BEHAVIOR
The Problem of Media Violence

According to a broad consensus of medical, public health, and government organizations, the evidence is now clear and convincing that exposure to media violence is *one* of the causal factors in real-life violence and aggression.[37] Of all media research, this is the one area that has been most thoroughly investigated. Research goes back as far as the 1950s,[38] and the US Senate held hearings on the subject in 1952. More than 2000 research reports are now listed by the new Center on Media and Child Health at Harvard.[39] A US Surgeon General's report in 1972,[40] a National Institute of Mental Health report 10 years later,[41] an FBI report on school shootings in 2000,[42] and most recently a Federal Communications Commission report in 2007[43] have all concluded that there is "strong evidence" that exposure to media violence can increase aggressive behavior in children and adolescents. More than 98% of pediatricians in one survey agree.[44] Yet the entertainment industry and a few professional naysayers have refused to accept these findings.[45] The debate should now be over.[46,47]

How Good Are the Data?

The strength of the association is sometimes at issue; certainly, media violence cannot be blamed as the leading cause of violence in society. But, epidemiologically, it does contribute approximately 10% to societal violence,[48] and the association between media violence and real-life violence is actually stronger than many of the public health risks that the public takes for granted (**Fig. 7**).

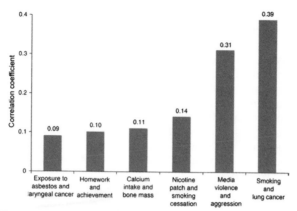

Fig. 7. The impact of media violence on real-life aggressive behavior is stronger than many commonly accepted public health risks and nearly as strong as the link between smoking and lung cancer. (*Adapted from* Bushman BJ, Huesmann LR. Effects of televised violence on aggression. In: Singer DG, Singer JL, editors. Handbook of children and the media. Thousand Oaks (CA): Sage; 2001; with permission.)

The research is also clear that nearly everyone is desensitized by the violence they witness vicariously, through the media,[49,50] and that media violence that seems acceptable to adults can be extremely scary for young children.[50,51]

"Old" Media

The problems with media violence are both quantitative and qualitative. In terms of quantity, American children and adolescents are inundated with portrayals of violence:

- The National Television Violence Study examined 10,000 hours of programming from 1995 to 1997 and found that 61% contained interpersonal violence. Counterintuitively, children's programming actually contained more violence than adult programming.[52]
- Similarly, children's films are rife with violence, even G-rated films. A study of all animated feature films between 1937 and 1999 found that 100% portrayed violence.[53]
- Films for preteens and teens are just as violent: a study of the top-rated PG-13 films of 1999–2000 found that 90% contained violence, half of it of lethal magnitude.[54] In 2003, more than 10% of 10- to 14-year-olds saw 40 of the most violent movies.[55]
- Several studies show that children can easily access violent media that their parents would deem inappropriate for them.[13,56] A recent analysis of the content of popular films from 1988 to 2006 found significant increases in violent content in the PG-13 rating category, leading the authors to conclude that there has been a greater leniency toward violent content by the Motion Picture Association of America ratings board.[57]
- Music lyrics have also become more violent, especially rap music.[58]

"New" Media

New technology has brought media violence into new platforms and into much more intimate settings, like children's bedrooms:

- A survey of 1500 10- to 15-year-olds found that 38% had been exposed to violent scenes on the Internet.[59]

- Half of all video games contain violence, including more than 90% of games rated appropriate for children 10 years or older (E10+ and T ratings).[60] Video games can mimic sexual assault ("RapeLay") or the Columbine massacre ("School Shooter"), allow the player to torture enemies ("Soldier of Fortune"), play "fetch" with dogs chasing the heads of slaughtered victims ("Postal 2"), cut victims in 2 from the crotch up with a chainsaw ("MadWorld"), or just brutally murder people ("Manhunt").
- Violent video games are also extremely popular, especially with boys. Children in the fourth to eighth grades prefer playing violent video games, and more than three-fourths of boys reported owning M-rated games in one survey.[61,62] Recent research suggests that playing violent games that feature violence against women is positively associated with Rape Myth Acceptance and negative attitudes toward women.[63]
- Cyberbullying has become a new and significant concern, although the magnitude of the problem is difficult to discern. Several reports put the figure at between 9% and 35% of young people who say that they have experienced electronic aggression.[64–69] Internet bullying may peak in middle school.[70] Rates of perpetration are lower in high school, 4%–21%.[65] The type of aggression varies from rude comments (32%) to threatening comments (14%) to rumors (13%).[66] As with other forms of bullying, there is overlap between victims and perpetrators, with 7% to 14% of youth reporting being both a victim and a perpetrator of electronic aggression.[66,71]
- Although some overlap exists, nearly two-thirds of 10- to 15-year-olds who say they were harassed online did not report being bullied at school. Of concern, youth who report being cyberbullied were 8 times more likely than all other youth to report carrying a weapon to school in the past 30 days.[65]
- A 3-year survey of more than 1500 10- to 15-year-olds from 2006 to 2008 has found an increase in text messaging harassment over time, with nearly 20% of the sample reporting harassment via text messaging in the previous year.[69]

Qualitatively, American media not only display violence frequently, but they do so in very problematic ways: funny violence,[72] justifiable violence,[52] realistic violence,[52] and violence without consequences.[52] The notion of "justifiable violence" ("good guys" vs "bad guys") is the most prevalent and the most positively reinforcing feature of American media violence.[37,45,73] Research has shown that repeated exposure to media violence can lead to anxiety and fear, particularly for young children,[51] acceptance of violence as a suitable means for resolving conflict,[74] desensitization,[49] and decreases in altruism.[75]

There are only a handful of studies to date on cyberbullying and its effects. For the perpetrators, it may be a strong predictor of serious aggressive behavior.[65,68] For the victims, the impact seems to be somewhat magnified because children and teens no longer feel safe at home, as they would with in-person bullying at school.[76]

New media have amplified the potential impact: variants of first-person shooter video games like "Manhunt" and "Call of Duty" are used by the US military to desensitize new recruits.[77] In one of the school shootings during the 1990s, a teenager walked into his school in Paducah, Kentucky, and opened fire on a prayer group. In spite of never having fired a gun in his life, Michael Carneal hit 8 different teens with 8 shots, all head and upper torso, resulting in 3 deaths and 1 case of paralysis. He had learned to fire a gun from playing first-person shooter video games.[77]

SEX

In the absence of effective sex education by parents or in schools, the media have arguably become the leading sex educator in the United States today.[78–80] Given how suggestive mainstream media content is, and how shy writers, producers, and advertisers are about depicting birth control, this is not an entirely healthy situation.[79] There is now considerable research that sexual content in the media contribute not only to adolescents' attitudes and beliefs about sex,[81] but to their sexual behavior as well, especially to earlier intercourse.[82] Although the teenage pregnancy rate in the United States has declined significantly in the past 2 decades, it remains the highest in the Western world.[83] In 2009, more than 400,000 15- to 19-year-olds gave birth: 4% of all female teens in that age group.[84] Also in 2009, nearly half of all high school students reported ever having had sexual intercourse.[85] Any factor that could possibly help delay intercourse among young teenagers, lower rates of sexually transmitted infections (STIs), or prevent pregnancy is worth considering.

Sexual Content in "Old" and "New" Media and Its Impact

Clearly, teenagers' use of media is in a state of flux; but it is equally clear that sexual content is now pervasive: TV, movies, magazines, music, Internet, video games, cell phones, and social networking sites. Unfortunately, the last major content analysis of American TV is now 6 years old.[86] At that time, more than 75% of primetime TV programs contained sexual content, yet only 14% of sexual references mentioned risks or responsibilities of sexual activity (**Fig. 8**). A newer study finds that although parents worry about exposure to sexual material on the Internet, TV is the leading culprit: exposure to sexual content is highest with TV (75%) compared with music (69%) and the Internet (16%–25%).[87] Research also shows that the amount of sexual content has continued to increase during the past 2 decades,[88,89] and remarkably, teen shows actually have more sexual content now than adult shows.[86] Talk about sex can occur as often as 8 to 10 times per hour.[88] Recently, so-called reality shows have become rife with sex; and the major theme seems to be who "hooks up" with whom.[79,89] In 1997, there were only 3 reality dating shows; by 2004, there were more than 30.

Examples of provocative teenage sex on TV are numerous: the MTV series *Skins* featured teen girls having sex with each other and teen boys taking erectile dysfunction drugs; CW's *Gossip Girl* has featured a threesome; and Showtime's *Shameless* depicts both teenage boys as being sexually active—one of them with a married man.[90] One survey actually found that in the 25 highest-rated primetime series among teenagers, teen female characters were engaged in sexual behavior 47% of the time versus adult women only 29% of the time.[91] Similarly, sexual language is flowing freely on primetime

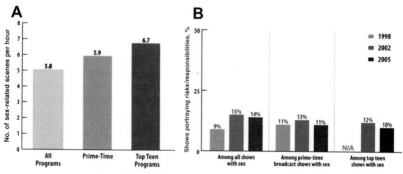

Fig. 8. (*A*) Programs for teenagers actually contain more sexual content than adult-oriented programs. (*B*) Despite the prevalence of sexual content on television, fewer than 14% of shows contain any mention of the risks and responsibility of sexual activity. (*Reproduced with permission from* Kaiser Family Foundation. Sex on TV 4, Executive Summary 2005. Available at: www.kff.org/entmedia/upload/sex-on-TV-Executive-Summary.pdf.)

TV. The 2011 Fall season has been termed "television's season of the vagina," with comments like "When did vaginas get so boring" on the new comedy *Whitney* and "that's the sound of my vagina drying up" on the hit comedy *Two Broke Girls*.[92,93] Yet, curiously, discussion of contraception remains rare among shows popular with teens. *Glee* never mentions birth control, one of the *Gossip Girl* characters has had sex with at least 8 different men without mention of contraception, and *90210* has had an HIV-positive storyline but rarely mentions safe sex. Only *The Secret Life of the American Teenager* has discussed both birth control pills and condoms and ends with a public service announcement (PSA) directing teens to health care resources.[94]

Other "old" media are also filled with sexual content:

- Pornography is a big business in the United States, nearly $13 billion a year,[95,96] and teenagers have surprisingly easy access to a variety of R- and X-rated material. In one 2001 study, 30% of teen girls had seen an X-rated movie within the prior 3 months.[97] Older studies have found that nearly all 13- to 15-year-olds report having seen an X-rated film and that by age 15, most teenagers have seen or read *Playboy*, *Playgirl*, or similar magazines.[8] Newer studies have found that the increased use of the Internet by teens has dramatically increased exposure to X-rated materials. Recent studies find that more than 50% of teens indicate exposure to "unwanted" sexual material.[97] Of concern is the fact that many popular pornographic videos depict aggression against women.[98]
- An analysis of the 279 most popular songs in 2005 showed that more than one-third contained sexual references, many of which were degrading to women.[99] A survey of the *Billboard Top 100* year-end songs at the end of every decade from 1959 to 2009 found significant increases in sexy lyrics.[100]
- Virtually *every* R-rated teen movie since the 1980s has contained at least 1 nude sex scene and often several references to sexual intercourse.[79]
- Teen magazines devote an average of 2.5 pages per issue to sexual topics, and the prime subject of discussion seems to be when to lose one's virginity.[81,101]
- In one study of mainstream advertising, women were as likely to be shown in suggestive clothing (30%), partially clothed (13%), or nude (6%) as they were being fully clothed.[102]

The question always asked of media researchers is, "does any of this abundant sexual content have any actual behavioral consequences?" Increasingly, the answer is yes. There are now 14 longitudinal correlational studies that allow cause-and-effect conclusions to be drawn,[82] and virtually all of them show an impact of sexual content in the media on adolescents' sexual behavior (**Table 1**).[103–119] In particular, the risk of early sexual intercourse appears to double with exposure to a lot of sexual content at a young age.[79,80] Exposure to degrading sexual lyrics has also been reported to be a risk factor for early sexual experience among teens.[120]

Contraceptive Advertising

One of the more intriguing aspects of media sex is that the entertainment industry is seemingly so fond of depicting sex but so reticent about discussing birth control.[121,122] The same applies to the advertising industry as well. Sex is used to sell virtually every product imaginable *except* for birth control. In particular, ads for erectile dysfunction (ED) drugs now dominate the TV screen. In the first 10 months of 2004, the makers of these drugs spent nearly $350 million on advertising.[123] By 2008, more drug company money was being spent on direct-to-consumer advertising ED drugs than on statins, antidepressants, bone resorption inhibitors, or sleep meds.[124]

The United States is the only Western country that still subscribes to the myth that giving teenagers access to birth control will make them sexually active at a younger age.[79] And the media now represent a major access point for teens about sex, sexuality, and contraception. Nine published, peer-reviewed studies have found that giving teenagers access to birth control does not increase their sexual activity but does increase their use of contraception and decreases their risk of sexually transmitted infections.[125–133] Yet several of the 6 major TV networks refuse to air ads for condoms or birth control pills.[79,122] In one well-publicized incident, both FOX and CBS refused to air an ad for Trojan condoms ("Evolve. Use a condom every time.") because those 2 networks will only air condom ads that restrict their content to preventing HIV and AIDS, not other STIs or pregnancy.[122] Ads for birth control pills are similarly rarely aired and when they are, the words "pregnancy-prevention" are nearly always absent.[79] Ads for emergency contraception are virtually nonexistent, yet every year American women have 3 million unplanned pregnancies, which lead to 1.3 million abortions. Advertising emergency contraception could be a major way to reduce the number of abortions in the United States.[134]

With "new" media have come not only the traditional concerns but a host of new concerns as well: easier exposure to pornography via the Internet, sexting, the posting of risky behaviors on social networking sites, and online solicitation for sex. Young people's exposure to online pornography is obviously difficult to assess accurately, given research restraints and the fact that studies have to rely on self-reports. A 2001 Kaiser Family Foundation survey found that 70% of teenagers had been exposed to pornography, although most of them said it had been "inadvertent."[135] A newer study of 1500 youth nationwide found that by 2006, only 42% reported seeing pornography online[136]; however, another recent study puts the figure at 93% of males and 62% of females by age 18.[137] As with X-rated movies and explicit magazines, it is entirely possible that most teenagers have seen online pornography by the time they finish high school.[97]

What impact pornography has on young people is conjectural at best, as researchers are prohibited from studying them in detail about such a sensitive subject. By necessity, nearly all studies on pornography and young people come from college-age students. Summarizing the vast adult literature is problematic,[138] but in general the research shows that nonviolent pornography has no behavioral consequences, but violent pornography, like media violence in general, may.[8] Only 4 studies have specifically examined children or teenagers:

- A recent longitudinal study of more than 1500 10- to 15-year-olds found a nearly sixfold increase in the odds of self-reported sexually aggressive behavior with exposure to violent x-rated material over time, whereas exposure to nonviolent x-rated material was not statistically related.[99]
- Another longitudinal study found that exposure to x-rated material (magazines, movies, and Internet porn) increased the risk of early sexual intercourse or oral sex.[113]
- A third study found an increase in "sexual preoccupation" with exposure to Internet pornography.[112]
- A cross-sectional study of 433 adolescents in New York City found that visiting sexually explicit Web sites was linked to a greater likelihood of having multiple lifetime sexual partners and having greater sexual permissiveness.[139]

Sexting

The dilemma of how to get accurate prevalence data is similar for "sexting"—the transmission via cell phone of sexually explicit photos.[140] The first study was done

Table 1
Recent longitudinal studies of the impact of sexual content on sexual behavior

Study	N	Media Type	Duration	Findings
Wingood et al,[103] 2003	480 14–18 y females	Rap videos	1 y	Exposure to sexual rap videos predicted multiple partners
Collins et al,[104] 2004	1792 12–17 y	TV	1 y	Sexual media exposure strongly predicted intercourse a year later
Ashby, et al,[105] 2006	4808 7th–12th grade	TV	1 y	>2 h TV/d increased risk of intercourse 1.35×
Brown et al,[106] 2006	1107 12–14 y	Sexual media, media diet (TV, movies, magazines, music)	2 y	2× increased risk of sexual intercourse for white teens with high sexual media diet
Martino et al,[107] 2006	1242 12–17 y	Music	3 y	Degrading sexual content predicted earlier intercourse
Bersamin et al,[109] 2008	887 12–16 y	TV	1 y	Parental co-viewing of TV protective against early intercourse and oral sex
Bleakley et al,[110] 2008	501 14–16 y	TV, movies, magazines, music, video games	1 y	Positive and reciprocal relationship between media exposure and intercourse
Chandra et al,[108] 2008	744 12–20 y	TV	3 y	Sexual media exposure = a strong predictor of teen pregnancy
Peter & Valkenburg,[111] 2008	962 13–20 y	Internet	1 y	Exposure to sexual content on the Internet increased sexual preoccupation
Brown and L'Engle,[112] 2009	967 7th–8th graders	X-rated movies magazines, Internet porn	2 y	Early exposure to X-rated media predicts earlier onset of sexual intercourse and oral sex

Study	N, Age	Media	Duration	Findings
Delgado et al,[113] 2009	754, 7–18 y	TV, movies	5 y	Watching adult-targeted TV increases the risk of intercourse by 33% for every h/d viewed at a young age
Hennessy et al,[114] 2009	506, 14–18 y	TV, movies, magazines, music, video games	2 y	Increased risk of intercourse for white teens and media
Bersamin et al,[115] 2010	824, 14–18 y	TV	1 y	Premium cable TV viewing associated with casual sex
Ybarra et al,[116] 2011	1159, 10–15 y	X-rated media (movies, magazines, Internet pornography)	3 y	Intentional exposure to violent X-rated material predicted a nearly 6× risk of sexually aggressive behavior
Martino et al,[117] 2005	1292, 12–17 y	TV	1 y	Exposure to popular teen shows with sexual content increased risk of intercourse 1 year later
L'Engle and Jackson,[118] 2008	854, 12–14 y	Sexual media diet	2 y	Peer and media exposure increased risk of early including Internet sex; Stronger connection to parents and schools was protective
Gottfried et al,[119] 2011	474, 14–16 y	TV-varying genres	1 y	No impact of overall sexual content found on sexual intercourse but exposure to TV sitcoms did predict earlier intercourse

by the National Campaign to Prevent Teen and Unplanned Pregnancy and found that 20% of nearly 1300 teens in a national survey had sent or posted nude or seminude pictures of themselves[141]; however, this study included 18- to 19-year-olds as well as younger teenagers. Much depends on (1) how the population is defined (Internet users versus all teens, although the 2 groups are becoming virtually the same), (2) how sexting is defined (is it sending photos, receiving them, or both?), and (3) what time period is under scrutiny (the past year or ever?). Since then, 5 more studies have been done, again with varying definitions of sexting and varying sample sizes and ages (**Table 2**).[14,142–145] The prevalence varies as well, especially when the difference between creating and sending explicit photos versus receiving them is ascertained. The "best guess" probably involves the 2 most recent studies. Both the Pew survey and the Youth Internet Safety Survey (YISS)-3 study found a relatively low prevalence of sending explicit messages and a slightly higher rate of receiving them. When the total number of young people online is considered, however, many experts feel that these figures are still alarming.[76] In addition, the legal consequences of sexting may be dire: several states have tried sexting teens as sexual offenders under child pornography laws.[146–148] Yet others have recognized that child pornography laws were initially passed to prevent childhood sexual abuse, not to keep teenagers, with their natural curiosity about sex, from doing dumb things.[149] States like New York and Vermont have moved to decriminalize sexting among teenagers, and other states have made it a misdemeanor rather than a felony. Finally, one new but related area of

Table 2
How prevalent is "sexting"?

Study	Sample	Prevalence	Definition
Sex Tech Survey (2008)	653 teens 13–19 y 627 20–26 y	20%	Sent or posted online nude or seminude pictures or videos
Harris/Teen Online (2009)	655 teens 13–18 y	19%	Received sexually suggestive text messages or e-mails with nude or nearly nude photos
		9%	Sent messages or e-mails
AP-MTV Survey (2009)	1247 14–24 y	45%	Sending or receiving nude or receiving nude photos of themselves or sexual partners via cell phone
South West Grid Survey (2009)	535 teens 13–18 y	40%	Students who knew friends who had shared "intimate" pix or videos
Pew Internet Project (2009)	800 teens 12–17 y	4%	Sent a sexually suggestive nude or seminude picture or video via cell phone
		9%	Received pix or video
Youth Internet Safety Survey 3 (YISS) 2011	1560 10–17 y	7.5%	Creating, appearing in, or receiving pictures showing breasts, genitals, or bottoms during the past year

Data from Strasburger VC. Adolescents, sex, and the media. Adolesc Med State Art Rev, in press.

concern is "sextortion"—threatening to send sexually explicit photos via e-mail or the Internet. Several high-profile cases have been prosecuted that have involved the victimization of teens, but no data currently exist on the prevalence of this.[150]

Social Networking

Research about social networking and sexual content is still very preliminary. A study of 270 profiles of 18-year-olds on MySpace found that 24% referenced sexual behaviors,[151] but of course MySpace has now been far outdistanced by Facebook. Adolescents who display explicit sexual references also have online friends who do likewise.[152] Among college freshmen, displaying sexual references on Facebook profile pages is positively correlated with intention to initiate intercourse.[153]

Online Solicitation

As with "sexting," reports vary considerably about the prevalence of online solicitations and even about the severity of it as a problem. Between 2000 and 2005, there was a decline in online sexual solicitations according to the first 2 YISS, from 27% of girls in 2000 to 18% in 2005.[154] In the 2007 Growing Up With Media Survey of more than 1500 10- to 15-year-olds, 15% reported an unwanted sexual solicitation online in the previous year. By 2008, this figure had increased to nearly 18%.[69] Only 4% were via a social networking site; more occurred through instant messaging and chat rooms.[155] An examination of more than 7000 arrests for Internet-related sex crimes against minors in 2006 had similar findings: one-third involved social networking sites, but the vast majority were via chat rooms or sting operations.[156] Teenage girls with a history of childhood abuse and provocative online avatars appear to be at increased risk.[157] But the conventional wisdom seems to be that online predatory crimes more often fit into the category of statutory rape by adult offenders with teenagers rather than forcible sexual assault or pedophilia.[158]

Prosocial sexual media

Although all of this sounds alarming and concerning, both "old" and "new" media can be a powerful source of positive sexual information as well. Storylines can feature depictions of responsible sexual activity (loving partners, use of birth control, and so forth), as well as useful health information. The hit show *ER* has dealt with the usefulness of contraception and the risks of human papillomavirus.[159] A 2002 *Friends* episode showed Rachel getting pregnant, despite Ross using a condom. Research by the Rand Corporation found that adolescents who talked about the program content with an adult were more likely to report learning about condoms from the episode and appeared less likely to reduce their perceptions of condom efficacy after the episode.[160] A 2008 episode of *Grey's Anatomy* successfully taught viewers that an HIV+ mother could deliver an HIV− baby.[161] Most recently, the hit show *Glee* has used the bullying of a gay teenager to dramatically sensitize viewers to both issues.[162] To date, shows like *The Secret Life of an American Teenager*, *Teen Mom*, and *16 and Pregnant* are more controversial; and their behavioral impact has not yet been rigorously evaluated[163]; however, in one survey of 162 10- to 19-year-olds, 93% responded that such shows teach them "that teen parenthood is harder than [they] imagined."[164]

Traditional sex education programs have been expanded to include media education topics and have been shown to be effective.[165] Finally, in North Carolina, a mass media campaign used billboards and radio and TV PSAs to deliver the message, "Talk to your kids about sex. Everyone else is." Exposure to the campaign message resulted in a significant increase in parents talking to their children about sex in the following month.[166]

New technology is also exploding with possibilities[6,167]:

- Text-messaging safe sex information[168] and information and results of testing for STIs[169]
- Using computer video games like "The Baby Game!" and "It's Your Game: Keep It Real" to increase knowledge and attitudes favoring avoiding teen pregnancy[170,171]
- New and potent sources of information about birth control, menstruation, pregnancy, and STIs, which may actually have a greater impact than health care providers or family (**Fig. 9**)
- Responsible online sites like Go Ask Alice, Sex, etc, Planned Parenthood, True Love Waits
- Using viral videos to encourage testing for HIV[172]
- Analogous to traditional media education, online media education about social networking sites has been shown to reduce displays of risky behaviors.[173]

SUBSTANCE USE AND ABUSE

As with aggressive behavior and sexual activity, the causes of adolescent drug use are multifactorial; but the media can and do often play a significant role.[174,175] In particular, alcohol and tobacco pose the greatest threat to young people and are also the

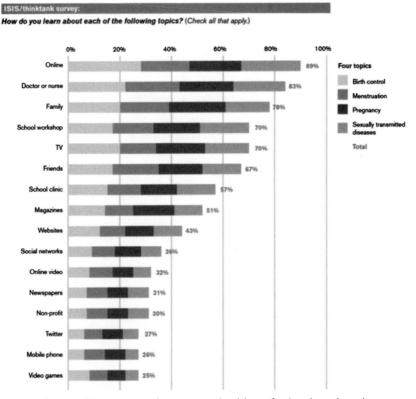

Fig. 9. Together, media now outrank parents or health professionals as the primary source of information about sex for teenagers. (*From* Boyar R, Levine D, Zensius N. TECHsex USA: youth sexuality and reproductive health in the digital age. Oakland (CA): ISIS, Inc.; April, 2011.)

most heavily advertised and depicted. Every year, more than 400,000 Americans die from tobacco-related causes—more than from AIDS, automobile accidents, murder, and suicide combined.[176] The substantial decrease in teen smoking that began in the mid-1990s appears to have come to a halt; nearly 20% of high school seniors have smoked cigarettes in the 30 days before being surveyed, and 42% of high school seniors have ever tried smoking.[177] Excessive alcohol consumption contributes to more than 100,000 deaths per year, including 5000 young people younger than 21.[178] By 12th grade, more than 70% of adolescents have used alcohol, and 54% have been drunk.[177] As for other drugs, 21% of 8th graders, 37% of 10th graders, and 48% of 12th graders have used an illicit substance, usually marijuana.[177]

Advertising

More than $20 billion a year is spent advertising and promoting tobacco, alcohol, and prescription drugs in the United States.[176] Big Tobacco spends the lion's share: an estimated $10 billion per year.[179] The Public Health Cigarette Smoking Act, which banned advertising on radio and television, went into effect in 1971. Many people forget that cigarette smoking ads were taken off of TV in the early 1970s, not because of tobacco's toll on society but because the tobacco lobby agreed to a ban.[175,180] It allowed cigarette manufacturers to put the money into marketing and promotion; advertise in alternative venues like stadiums, magazines, and billboards; and resulted in the disappearance of antismoking ads on TV. Given the demographics of smoking (1200 deaths per day, 50% of smokers begin by age 13 and 90% by age 19) it is imperative for the industry to recruit new, young smokers.[181] Specific age and ethnic groups are often targeted. For example, the Camel No. 9 advertising campaign in 2007 seemed custom-made for young teenage girls and was very effective.[182]

What impact does cigarette advertising still have, given that it is no longer on TV or radio? A meta-analysis of 51 separate studies found that exposure to tobacco marketing and advertising more than doubles the risk of a teenager beginning to smoke.[183] In 1994, the US Surgeon General concluded that cigarette advertising increases young people's risk of smoking,[181] and the fact that the most heavily advertised brands are also the most popular would seem to confirm that.[184] Magazines popular with teenagers have attracted an increasing number of cigarette ads since 1965.[185] Numerous studies have shown that children or teens who pay closer attention to cigarette ads or who own promotional items are more likely to become smokers

Table 3
How good is the research linking tobacco marketing to onset of adolescent smoking?

Research Question	No. of Studies	No. of Subjects Studied
Are nonsmoking children exposed to and more aware of tobacco promotion? YES	4 prospective 12 cross-sectional	37,649
Does exposure to promotions increase the risk of initiation? YES	12 prospective 14 cross-sectional 2 time-series	349,306
Does a dose-response relationship exist? YES	2 prospective 7 cross-sectional	25,180

Data from Strasburger VC, Council on Communications and Media. Media violence (policy statement). Pediatrics 2010;124;1495–503; and DiFranza JR, Wellman RJ, Sargent JD, et al. Tobacco Consortium, Center for Child Health Research of the American Academy of Pediatrics. Tobacco promotion and the initiation of tobacco use: assessing the evidence for causality. Pediatrics 2006;117(6):e1237–48.

themselves.[186–188] The research is clear and convincing (**Table 3**).[175,176] The Family Smoking Prevention and Tobacco Control Act imposes new warnings and labels on tobacco packaging and their advertisements.[189] The 9 new warning labels that cigarette makers have to use on their packaging have not yet been put into effect, and are already being challenged by US tobacco companies as violating their free speech rights (**Fig. 10**).

Approximately $5 billion a year is spent on alcohol advertising and promotion.[190] As with tobacco ads, alcohol ads seem "custom-made" to attract children and adolescents: funny scenes, sexy models, talking animals (**Fig. 11**).[175,191] Unlike tobacco advertising, alcohol advertising faces few restrictions, and young people see an average of 2000 ads annually.[192] Between 2001 and 2009, teenagers were actually exposed to more alcohol advertising on TV than adults: an increase of 71%, largely because of the advertising of distilled spirits and the presence of alcohol ads on programs popular with teenagers.[193,194] This has occurred despite the industry's 2003 promise to advertise only when the underage audience comprises less than 30% of the total viewing audience. Young people are 22 times more likely to see an alcohol ad than a "responsibility" ad warning against underage drinking or impaired driving.[193] On the other hand, the industry also pledged to observe the same 30% figure with magazine advertising, and from 2001 to 2008 it did achieve that goal: adolescent exposure to alcohol advertising in magazines decreased by 48%.[195] Many studies have shown that exposure to alcohol advertising results in more positive beliefs about drinking and is predictive of underage drinking.[196–201]

Many experts feel that prescription drug advertising also contributes to adolescent drug use.[176,202] Children and teenagers get the clear message that there is a pill to cure all ills, a pill for every occasion (even sexual intercourse). Nearly $4 billion annually is spent on prescription drug advertising,[203] and drug companies now spend more than twice as much money on marketing as they do on research and development.[204] The United States and New Zealand are the only countries in the world that allow prescription drugs to be advertised.

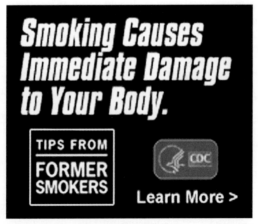

Fig. 10. The FDA is trying to experiment with new and more graphic cigarette package labels, and the CDC is initiating a more graphic public health campaign. The FDA's efforts are being vigorously opposed by the tobacco industry. The proposed new labels are available at: http://www.fda.gov/TobaccoProducts/Labeling/ucm259214.htm#High_Resolution_Image_Formats. (*From* US food and Drug Administration. tobacco products: labeling. Available at: http://www.fda.gov/TobaccoProducts/Labeling/default.htm.)

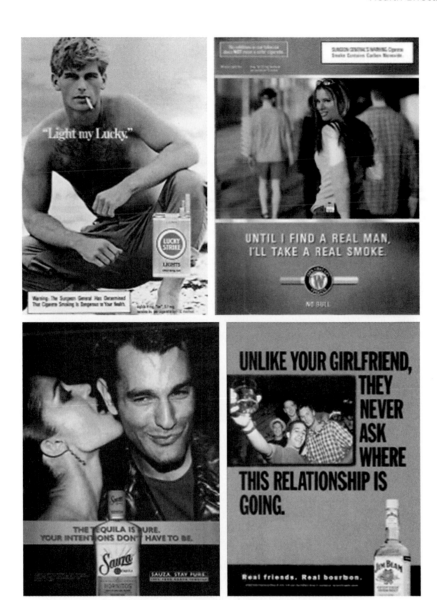

Fig. 11. Tobacco and alcohol ads seem custom-made to attract teenagers. Such ads make smoking cigarettes and drinking alcohol seem like normative behavior.

Drugs in Entertainment Media

Regarding smoking in the movies, there is both good news and bad news. The good news is that smoking in the movies is decreasing. A number of studies in the late 1990s and early 2000s had documented that most movies popular with teenagers contained images of smoking.[205,206] Even G-rated movies for young children were found to be rife with smoking.[207] But the latest content analyses shows that since 2005, there has been a decline[208,209]: the percentage of all top-growing movies that did not show tobacco use exceeded 50% for the first time in 2009.[209] The bad news is that in 2009, more than half of PG-13 movies still contained scenes of tobacco use,[209] and research is now showing that exposure to scenes of movie smoking may be the leading predictor of young teens' initiation of smoking (**Fig. 12**).[210–217] Young people who witness a lot of movie smoking are 2 to 3 times more likely to begin smoking.[212] Some researchers estimate that more than half of all smoking initiation is caused by exposure to smoking in movies.[210,213] Preteens whose parents forbid them from seeing R-rated movies are less likely to begin smoking (or drinking).[17,218] Those who study adolescent risk-taking argue the importance of understanding parenting styles, including monitoring behaviors in general, to understand children's access to media and time spent with media.[219]

Viewing scenes of smoking on TV may fall into the same category as viewing smoking in the movies, although there are no longitudinal studies yet to prove this. A content analysis of top-rated TV shows for teenagers during the fall 2007 season did show that 40% of TV shows had at least 1 depiction of tobacco use, resulting in nearly 1 million youth exposed to smoking scenes for the shows that were studied.[220] Movie trailers shown on TV are also a rich source of smoking scenes,[221] and one study has shown that such trailers increase the attractiveness of smoking among teens who have already experimented with cigarettes.[222]

Alcohol remains the number 1 drug portrayed on American television, however. A study of the top 10 TV shows from 2004 to 2006 found that one-third of episodes examined featured alcohol use.[223] On MTV, teenagers can see alcohol use every 14 minutes.[224] Teens who typically watch popular teen reality shows like *Jersey Shore*,

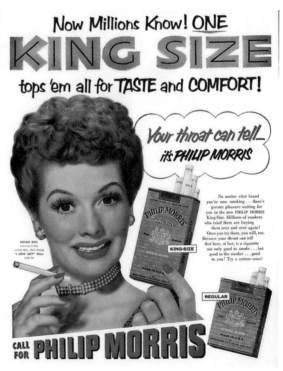

Fig. 12. Movie star smoking has always glamorized smoking for children, teenagers, and adults. Many old-time movie stars (eg, Lucille Ball, John Wayne, James Dean, Humphrey Bogart) smoked onscreen and off. Research studies now show that viewing scenes of movie smoking is one of the key factors in the onset of adolescent smoking.[207–217]

Teen Mom, *16 and Pregnant*, or teen dramas like *Skins* or *Gossip Girl* were nearly twice as likely to use alcohol in one recent national survey of more than1000 teenagers.[225] Popular music is also a source of alcohol references, especially rap music. From 1979 to 1997, songs with alcohol references increased from 8% to 44%.[58] Popular movies are also filled with alcohol use; only 2 of the 40 highest-grossing movies in one study did not contain scenes of alcohol use.[226] Again, the impact from the research is clear: exposure to scenes of drinking in mainstream media is strongly predictive of drinking onset and binge drinking in adolescents.[194,227–229]

Movies are powerful influences: one study found that teenagers who watch more than 3 R-rated films per month are 5 times more likely to drink alcohol than teens who watched none[230]; and in one intriguing study, 2- to 6-year-olds who were asked to shop in a make-believe store were 5 times more likely to buy beer or wine if they had been allowed to see PG-13 or R-rated movies.[231] The research includes correlational studies,[199,227] experimental studies,[231,232] and longitudinal studies.[197,226–229] As with media violence and sex in the media, *context matters*. In the case of alcohol (and other drugs), popular teen TV shows and movies invariably show drug use as being socially acceptable and consequence-free, and most characters are not even given the choice of whether to accept or reject the drugs being offered.[233]

Despite public perceptions, illegal drugs are rarely shown on TV, with the exception of cable shows like Showtime's *Weeds* (marijuana) and AMC's *Breaking Bad* (methamphetamine).[234] Even in movies, illicit drugs are not all that common, other than marijuana, which seems to be making a comeback in R-rated movies like the *Harold and Kumar* series, *Pineapple Express* (2008), *Due Date* (2010), and *Bad Teacher* (2011).[235] A Columbia University study found that viewing R-rated movies was associated with a sixfold increased risk of trying marijuana.[230] Hollywood filmmakers do not seem to understand that movies can function as a "super-peer" for teens[33] and that humor tends to undermine normal adolescent defenses against drugs and legitimizes their use.[175] Similarly, teens who listen to a lot of music are exposed to lyrics about marijuana. In one study of nearly 1000 ninth graders, the average listener heard 27 marijuana references per day; those most heavily exposed were more likely to have used marijuana.[236]

Research on the possible impact of new media on adolescent drug use is just beginning and mostly consists of content analyses. A study of all Web pages viewed by 346 14- to 17-year-olds during a 30-day period found that of the 1.2 million pages they viewed, 1916 pages had protobacco content, 1572 had antitobacco content, and 5055 pages had indeterminate content. Most of the tobacco content was found on social networking sites.[237] A content analysis of 400 randomly selected MySpace profiles discovered that 56% contained references to alcohol.[238] In a qualitative study, teens acknowledge that this constitutes a potential type of peer pressure.[239] Teens can also buy alcohol online,[240] but effective in October 2012, the Food and Drug Administration (FDA) must issue regulations to prevent the sale of tobacco products to underage youth online. One new correlational study suggests further research is needed: compared with teens who spend no time on social networking sites, teens who do were found to be 5 times likelier to use tobacco, 3 times likelier to use alcohol, and twice as likely to use marijuana.[225] Even more concerning, 40% of more than 1000 teens surveyed nationwide reported seeing pictures of kids getting drunk, passed out, or using drugs on social networking sites.[225]

OBESITY

In the 2011 National Poll on Children's Health, obesity was the number 1 health problem that parents worry about.[241] Given the current epidemic of obesity, not just in the United States but worldwide, any factor that might influence obesity would seem to be well worth investigating. Obesity represents a clear danger to the health and well-being of children and adolescents. When the producers of *Taking Woodstock* began casting for their movie about the 1969 concert, they had great difficulty finding extras who were as thin as the original concert-goers.[242] The prevalence of obesity has doubled in the past 3 decades, and there are now more overweight and obese adults in the United States than normal-weight adults.[243] Rates of obesity are increasing in nearly every country.[244] Global diabetes rates have doubled from 1980 to 2008; an estimated 350 million people worldwide now have diabetes.[245] The cost to American society is an estimated $168 billion a year, which is nearly 17% of all medical costs.[246]

The Role of Media

Considerable research is now finding that screen time plays an important role in the etiology of obesity.[247,248] A remarkable number of long-term studies in various countries are particularly persuasive, finding a connection even when all other known factors contributing to obesity are controlled for:

- Researchers in Dunedin, New Zealand, followed 1000 subjects from birth to 26 years of age and found that average weeknight TV viewing between the ages of 5 and 15 was strongly predictive of adult body mass index (BMI).[249]
- A 30-year study in the United Kingdom found that a higher mean of daily hours of TV viewed on weekends predicted a higher BMI at age 30, and for each additional hour of weekend TV watched at age 5, the risk of adult obesity increased 7%.[250]
- A study of 8000 Scottish children found that viewing more than 8 hours of TV per week at age 3 was associated with an increased risk of obesity at age 7.[251] Similarly, a study of 8000 Japanese children found that TV viewing at age 3 resulted in a higher risk of overweight at age 6.[252]

Large cross-sectional studies from both the United States[253–259] and other countries[260–263] have found similar results, although 1 US study and 1 Chinese study have suggested that TV advertising rather than programming is what contributes to obesity.[257,264] The presence of a bedroom TV exacerbates the problem, sometimes even independently of physical activity level.[16,265–268] One study found that teenagers with a bedroom TV spent more time watching TV, less time being physically active, ate fewer family meals, and consumed unhealthier diets than teens without a bedroom TV.[266] Studies have also found a link between excessive screen time and hypercholesterolemia,[269] hyperinsulinemia,[270] insulin resistance,[271] type 2 diabetes,[272] metabolic syndrome,[271,273] hypertension,[274] and even early mortality.[275]

So the connection between screen time and obesity is clear, but the exact reasons why are not. Possible mechanisms include (1) increased sedentary activity along with displacement of more active pursuits, (2) the impact of food advertising on children's food and beverage choices, (3) unhealthy eating behaviors while watching TV and learned from TV, and (4) interference with normal sleep patterns.

Sedentary Activities

One would think that the *displacement effect* (ie, if a child is sitting passively in front of a TV set or computer screen, he or she is not outside playing) might play a key role, but the research is conflicted on this point. Many studies have found that physical activity decreases as screen time increases,[256,276] but other studies have not.[277,278] A recent study of more than 72,000 schoolchildren from 34 countries found that nearly one-third are spending 3 hours a day or more watching TV or on the computer.[279] The problem could be that sedentary children and teenagers may remain sedentary even if screen time is not an option,[278,280,281] or that researchers' measures of physical activity may be too imprecise.[282] Nevertheless, the reverse seems to hold true: decreasing screen time does help to prevent obesity.[283–285] Several studies have looked at newer video games that involve exercise and seem to offer some hope (eg, *Dance Dance Revolution* and *Wii Sports*).[286–288] Energy expenditure during these games is equivalent to moderately paced walking.[289]

Food Advertising

In 2009, the fast-food industry alone spent $4.2 billion on advertising.[290] More than 80% of all ads in children's programming are for fast food or snacks.[291,292] Young people see an average of 12 to 21 food ads per day (4400–7600 ads per year), yet fewer than 165 ads that promote fitness or good nutrition.[293] Movies may also be a "hidden" source of product placements for unhealthy foods: in a study of 200 movies from 1996 to 2005, researchers found that 69% contained at least 1 food, a total of 1180 product placements were identified, and most of them were for energy-dense, nutrient-poor snacks.[294] Increasingly, online advergames (**Fig. 13**) and advertising are targeting young children as well.[295,296] A study of the top 5 brands of food and beverages found that all had Internet Web sites, 63% had advergames, 50% used cartoon characters, and 58% had a designated children's area.[297] Fewer than 3% of the games actually educate children about nutrition,[298] yet this could be a creative use of new technology to promote healthier food choices.[299]

The research is clear that children and teens who watch a lot of TV tend to consume more calories, eat higher-fat diets, drink more sodas, and eat fewer fruits and vegetables.[257,300] Perhaps the most intriguing study to document the effectiveness of food advertising involved 63 children who tasted 5 pairs of identical foods and beverages (eg, French fries, carrots, milk) from unbranded packaging versus McDonald's packaging. The children strongly preferred the McDonald's foods and drinks, even though all of the food and drinks were absolutely identical.[301]

In 2011, a working group comprising the Centers for Disease Control and Prevention, FDA, US Department of Agriculture, and Federal Trade Commission was convened to establish voluntary guidelines for marketing food to children.[302] The guidelines produced cover a wide array of marketing, from television to toys in fast food meals to Internet sites and social media and would severely limit advertising of foods that exceeded limited amounts of added sugar, saturated or trans fats, and sodium.[303] So far, food manufacturers have rejected the proposed guidelines in favor of their own, weaker guidelines.[303] It is highly debatable whether self-regulation will work in a multibillion-dollar industry that relies so heavily on child and adolescent consumption of unhealthy foods.[304–306]

Snacking Behavior

Some research suggests that viewing TV while eating actually suppresses satiety cues, leading to overeating.[307] Several studies have documented that eating while viewing leads to unhealthy practices:

- A study of 5000 Midwest middle and high school students found that high TV use is associated with more snacking and consumption of soda and fast food.[308]
- Similar studies of more than 162,000 preteens and teens in Europe correlated TV viewing with increased snacking.[309]

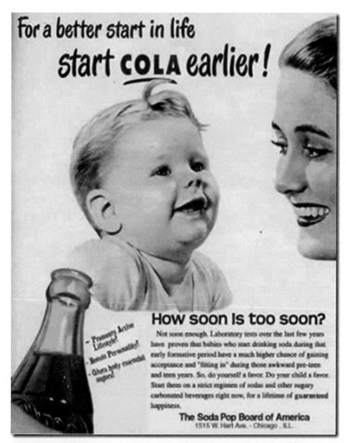

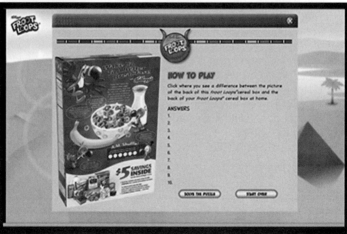

Fig. 13. (*Top*) Increased consumption of soda has contributed to the problem of obesity. (*Bottom*) Online advergames are increasingly popular with young children.

- A longitudinal study of 564 middle school students and 1366 high school students found that TV viewing predicted poorer dietary intake five years later.[310] (Barr-Anderson, 2009)
- Even experimental studies show this effect: a study of college students found that they take in an additional 163 kcal/day when they watch TV.[311]
- In a study of 548 students in 5 public schools near Boston, researchers found that each hour increase in TV viewing resulted in an additional 167 kcal/day being consumed.[312]

Other research suggests that viewers make unhealthy food choices because of the ads that they see, not the content of TV programming.[257,313] A prospective study of 827 third graders followed for 20 months found that total TV time predicted future requests for advertised foods and drinks.[314]

Sleep

One of the newest areas of research involves the impact of sleep on a variety of different health concerns, including obesity.[315–317] For example, a longitudinal study of young children in the United Kingdom found that shorter sleep duration at age 30 months predicted obesity at 7 years.[318] Significantly, several studies have now implicated TV viewing with a loss of sleep.[319,320] A longitudinal study of adolescents in New York found that viewing 3 or more hours per day of TV doubled the risk of difficulty falling asleep compared with watching less than 1 hour per day.[319] Later bedtimes and less sleep may be associated with a greater risk of obesity.[315,318] Again, the mechanisms are unclear: sleep loss may lead to increased snacking,[321] fatigue and increased sedentary activity,[322] or metabolic changes.[323] It is also possible that the light of a bedroom TV screen at night may interfere with melatonin release, which, in turn, interferes with sleep.[324]

BODY IMAGE AND EATING DISORDERS

A new report on eating disorders has found that hospitalizations surged 119% between 1999 and 2006 for children younger than 12.[325] Especially for girls, the media may play a crucial role in the formation of young people's body self-image; may be responsible for creating unrealistic expectations, body dissatisfaction; and may even contribute to the development of eating disorders.[326–329] For example, a large study of nearly 7000 9- to 14-year-olds found that girls who want to look like TV or movie stars were twice as likely to be concerned about their weight, to be constant dieters, or to engage in purging behavior.[330] For preteen and teenage girls, fashion and beauty magazines are particularly adept at displaying role-models with impossibly thin bodies (**Fig. 14**).[331] A study of nearly 3000 Spanish 12- to 21-year-olds over a 19-month period found that those who read girls' magazines had a doubled risk of developing an eating disorder.[332] A longitudinal study of 315 preteens found that TV exposure significantly predicted disordered eating a year later for girls.[333] And teenage girls on the Pacific island of Fiji had virtually no problems with eating disorders until American TV shows were introduced. Two years later, 75% of the teen girls surveyed reported feeling "too big or fat" and 15% had abnormal Eating Inventory scores.[334]

New media are contributing to this problem as well. There are now more than 100 pro-anorexia Web sites (pro-ana sites) that not only encourage disordered eating but offer specific advice on purging, severely restricting caloric intake, and exercising excessively.[335] And a follow-up study in Fiji found that social network media exposure was associated with eating pathology in a sample of 523 young girls.[336] Clearly, the media can and do play a crucial role in the development of body self-image.[326]

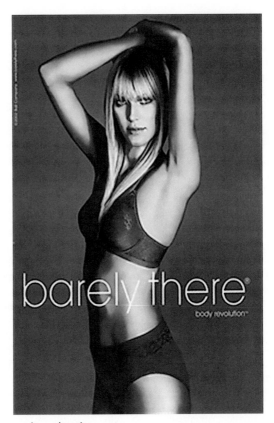

Fig. 14. Fashion magazine advertisement.

Although there are insufficient data to state that the media *cause* eating disorders, media exposure can certainly be considered as a significant risk factor.[337]

OTHER CONSIDERATIONS

Many other aspects of media's impact on child and adolescent health have been studied. In most cases, the samples studied are correlational and not longitudinal. Hence, associations can be inferred but not causation.

Infant Media

There are now at least 14 studies implicating infant screen time with language delays[338–351] and no studies conclusively showing that exposure to TV or infant videos alone for babies younger than 2 years accelerates their learning.[352] Only 2 studies thus far have shown new word acquisition from viewing TV or infant videos, and this was likely because of the influence of co-viewing by parents.[353,354] The most likely explanation is that the infant brain is "plastic" and responds to environmental stimuli, parents being the most important, by far; but also babies can discriminate between live human beings and actors on-screen.[355]

Attention-Deficit Disorder

Several studies have raised the possibility of a connection between TV viewing and attention-deficit disorder (ADD) or other learning problems.[356–358] The initial study in

2001 found an association between daily hours of TV viewing at ages 1 to 2 years and subsequent attention problems at age 7.[359] One subsequent study found the opposite: that healthy children demonstrate more cognitive impairment after watching TV than children with ADD.[359] A recent study also found that young autistic children watch more TV than other children.[360] This is currently a hot topic of investigation, and no cause-and-effect conclusions are possible yet; however, it is possible to conclude that excessive screen time and the presence of a bedroom TV have a negative impact on academic performance.[361–367]

Depression and Suicide

Studies have linked media coverage of and portrayals of suicide with an increase in actual suicides, a type of "suicide contagion" that affects teens far more than adults.[368–370] Even sensitively made-for-TV movies have resulted in an increase.[368,369] The Centers for Disease Control and Prevention actually issued guidelines in 2003 for reporting suicide in the media, which asks TV stations and newspapers to avoid sensationalizing suicides (eg, Kurt Cobain) or glorifying the person involved.[371]

Although no recent studies have been found involving TV or movies, major publicity now surrounds suicides precipitated by Internet bullying.[371,372] Excessive media use may also be a marker for depression[373] and has been associated with increased psychological distress in children and preteens.[374–378]

THE POSITIVE ROLE OF MEDIA IN THE LIVES OF CHILDREN AND ADOLESCENTS

Although much of this article has focused on research emphasizing the deleterious consequences of inappropriate and excessive media use, it is also critical to acknowledge the many positive roles media can play in children's healthy development (**Fig. 15**). A 1986 meta-analysis of studies investigating the effects of television on children concluded that positive effects of prosocial TV viewing were twice as strong and more enduring than antisocial effects of violent TV.[379] An update of the meta-analysis, conducted in 2005 with research released since the original study, also found consistently positive effects of prosocial content on children's behavior.[380] Videogames have also produced positive prosocial outcomes. In one experiment, college students who were assigned to play prosocial games were more helpful and less hurtful to a partner in a puzzle task, relative to those who played neutral or violent games.[63] A longitudinal survey conducted with 5th-, 8th-, and 11th-grade students in Japan found that students who played more prosocial games initially reported more prosocial behaviors 4 months later.[63]

Although heavy media use is implicated in obesity, relatively new products have created an opportunity to combine exercising with gaming. "Exergames" offer children and adolescents opportunities to engage in home-based exercise; and many schools have designed physical education classes around them. Although it is not yet clear whether games like *Dance Dance Revolution* or *Wii Fit* can be effective in weight loss,[381,382] there does seem to be some potential to use games as a positive force for health.[383] In one small study, 14 adolescents, 15 young adults, and 13 older adults were brought to a laboratory to compare the physiologic cost and enjoyment of playing an exergame (*Wii Fit*), a handheld inactive video game, and brisk treadmill walking and jogging. As might be expected, the physiologic cost of exergaming on *Wii Fit* was significantly greater than handheld inactive video gaming but lower than treadmill exercise. However, as the authors point out: "the acute enjoyment response derived from Wii balance and Wii aerobics was comparable if not greater than handheld inactive

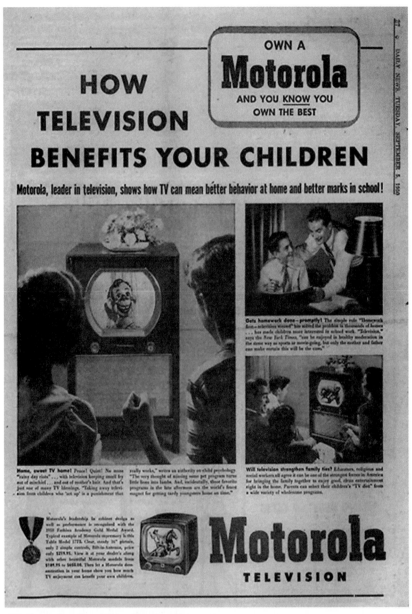

Fig. 15. Example of positive role advertisement.

gaming and treadmill exercise, especially in adolescents, suggesting individuals may be more likely to adhere to sustained light to moderate intensity exergaming."[384(p399)]

Media, if used properly, can introduce children to education and learning even when they come from families with very few resources. *Sesame Street*, which is perhaps the world's most carefully studied show, was designed to close the "knowledge gap" between children who have the financial resources to attend preschool and those who do not.[339] It has been wildly successful both in reaching its target audience of at-risk preschoolers but also in setting the standard for careful formative and summative research to track the program's effectiveness.[339] A longitudinal study tracking children from preschool through high school found that children who viewed *Sesame Street* and other educational preschool programs arrived at school more "ready to learn" and that these gains persisted through high school, even after controlling for individual and family variables that are known to affect educational success.[385] Another well-known television program, *Blue's Clues*, was designed to focus on preschoolers' cognitive problem solving. In a 2-year program evaluation, researchers followed preschoolers who were regular viewers of the show and preschoolers who were not because the program did not air in their town of residence. The 2 groups were equivalent in their problem solving at the start of the study. But at the end of the 2-year period, regular viewers of *Blue's Clues* outperformed their nonviewing peers in many measures, and were more successful and systematic in their problem solving.[386]

New media technologies give youth the opportunity to create their own expressions of individuality, whether through social networks like Facebook or file-sharing sites like YouTube.[7] In her research on adolescent use of social networks, danah boyd explains that "teens are drawn to social media collectively and ... individuals choose to participate because their friends do. The appeal is not technology itself—nor any particular technology, but the presence of friends and peers."[387(pp294–295)] New media allow adolescents to experience community in a time of life when they often feel unmoored. The It Gets Better Project, a Web site created after a series of suicides by youth who had been bullied over their sexuality, gives lesbian, gay, bisexual, and transgender (LGBT) youth the space to tell their stories and to hear the encouragement of LGBT adults who have successfully navigated the turbulent teen years (http://www.itgetsbetter.org/). As media experts Heather Kirkorian, Ellen Wartella, and Dan Anderson conclude "The influences can be both for good and for ill. ... Ultimately, however, the question is whether society has the ability and will to enhance the positive aspects of media and reduce the negative."[388(p54)]

SOLUTIONS

The potential for media to play a beneficial role in the lives of children and youth has not been fully realized, and strategies for reducing the negative effects have not been optimized. Clearly, children and adolescents learn from the media (**Fig. 16**).

PARENTS

For years, the American Academy of Pediatrics[389] (AAP) has recommended that parents

1. Limit total screen time for children older than 2 years to no more than 1 to 2 hours per day
2. Avoid screen time for children younger than 2 years
3. Keep children's bedrooms free of screen media (including TVs, computers, iPads, cell phones)
4. Co-view media with their children and teenagers and discuss the content.

Parental efforts to interpret, elaborate, and provide supplemental information on topics introduced by television have been found to be successful in countering negative or harmful content.[6] As the AAP states,[80] co-viewing with children and teens can effectively replace "the big talk" about sex and drugs. Although 65% of 1000 parents surveyed nationally in a recent study reported that they "closely monitor" their

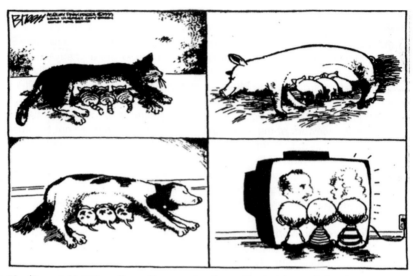

Fig. 16. (Copyright © Steve Breen/Creators Syndicate. Used with permission.)

children's media habits,[390] parents typically report that their children use less media than children themselves report.[391] Therefore, an important first step would be for health care providers to encourage parents to be more cognizant about their children's media time. Parents should be told why the AAP recommends limited time with screen media and emphasize the value of play for babies and toddlers, the importance of family dinners with the TV off, and the importance of unstructured time so that young children's imagination and creativity will be stimulated. A recent study found that interventions targeting the preschool age group might be most effective.[392] Parents also need to avoid exposing young children to PG-13– and R-rated movies,[229,393,394] and should set clear guidelines for online activities. As a corollary, parents should be mindful of their own media practices, as studies have shown that the strongest predictor of children's heavy media use is parents' heavy media use.[391,395]

For new technology, The AAP has launched a new parent-oriented Web site (http://www.healthychildren.org/English/family-life/Media/Pages/default.aspx) that provides suggestions for parents in dealing with topics as diverse as cyberbullying, food ads on TV, and media education. A recent clinical report from the AAP also advises parents to do the following[396]:

- Talk to their children and adolescents about their online use and the specific issues involved (eg, cyberbullying, sexting, advergames, and so forth)
- Become better educated about the many new technologies young people have access to
- Supervise their children's online activities directly, as opposed to remote monitoring with "Net-nanny"-type programs.

PRACTITIONERS

Because the media potentially have an impact on virtually *every* concern that parents and pediatricians have about children and adolescents, from aggressive behavior, early sexual activity, substance abuse, obesity, to school performance, a minute or 2 of counseling on media use would be time well spent. Yet a 2004 survey of 365 pediatricians revealed that only half recommend limiting screen time according to the AAP recommendations, and half said they were not interested in learning more about media influences on their patients.[44] One study found that just a minute or 2 of office counseling could result in nearly 1 million children adhering to the AAP guidelines of 2 hours of screen time per day.[397] Clinicians who see children need to understand that discussing children's media use may be as helpful to children's healthy development as explaining the importance of a bicycle helmet or the positioning of a car seat, particularly if a child is showing signs of school difficulty, aggressiveness, disordered eating, or poor sleep patterns. The following 2 questions are useful to pose to parents in the clinical setting:

1. How much time per day does the child or teenager spend with entertainment media?
2. Is there a television set or any electronic device that allows an Internet connection in the child's bedroom?[398,399]

Parents should be encouraged to avoid putting electronic devices in the child's bedroom to begin with or to remove them once they are there. For households with teenagers, the computer with an Internet connection is best placed in a living room or den where there is heavy adult traffic. Traditionally, continuing medical education programs for physicians have been planned along subspecialty lines; however, given that the media have an impact on virtually every concern that clinicians and parents have about children and adolescents, physicians need more information about media effects, such as the impact on teenage sex, drug use, suicide, and school achievement. In February, 2012, the American Academy of Pediatrics announced that Children, Adolescents, and Media would become part of its Strategic Plan for the next 2–3 years.

SCHOOLS

Schools have not kept pace with modern media, especially in violence prevention, drug prevention, and sex education programs. With the amount of sexual suggestiveness currently displayed on television and in movies, schools no longer have any excuse for not providing comprehensive school-based sex education programs for children and adolescents, including full discussions of contraception[400] and how sex and sexuality are portrayed in the media. Similarly, drug education programs must progress beyond scare tactics to incorporate principles of media education, teaching young people how to deconstruct alcohol and tobacco ads, and, thereby, become more resilient. Media education is now crucial. A century ago, to be "literate" meant that one could read and write; in 2009 it means having the ability to decipher a bewildering array of media and make sense of them all. Several countries, including the United Kingdom, Canada, and Australia, mandate such education in their schools.[401] Few American schools teach media education, but studies have shown that it may be useful in mitigating harmful media effects.[165,173,390,401–404] Even the use of new technologies can be affected through media education; one study revealed that teenagers can be responsive to messages about the dangers of posting sexual references in their profiles on social networking sites, for example, and will alter their online behavior accordingly.[173] Schools need to develop programs to educate young people about how to use new technology wisely, as well as school policies to deal with cyberbullying and sexting.[405]

ENTERTAINMENT INDUSTRY

Given the tremendous positive potential of mass media to provide millions of people with accurate and important health information, the entertainment industry must become more public health oriented than it currently is. The United States continues to have the highest teenage pregnancy rate in the Western world.[83] Given this fact, increasing responsible sexual content in mainstream media and advertising contraceptives widely would seem to be an urgent public health goal.[81] Several studios have agreed to add antismoking advertisements before feature films on new DVDs, and Disney no longer permits smoking in its movies.[406] Industry ratings systems have sometimes been confusing for parents, although most have indicated that they rely on the information.[390] For example, several national surveys of parents revealed that only 10% of parents understand that the television rating "FV" indicates "fantasy violence."[8,395] One major help for parents would be a universal ratings system for all media instead of the "alphabet soup" that currently exists separately for television, movies, and video games.[8]

ADVERTISING INDUSTRY

Currently, the United States spends $250 billion per year on advertising,[407] yet advertisers continue to claim that they are only trying to influence brand choice, not consumption. There are good data that show that advertising does increase consumer spending by children (AAP) and the products most advertised to children may not be the healthiest for them (eg, junk food and fast food),[408] whereas other products are woefully underadvertised (eg, healthy foods, contraceptives).[81,408,409] Given the new potential of digital advertising to reach an increasingly younger audience, it seems vital to establish appropriate advertising ethics for what can and cannot be advertised to certain age groups.[296] In particular, with the epidemic of obesity now spreading worldwide, some experts have suggested that limits be placed on advertising junk food and sugary beverages to children and adolescents,[300,410–412] a move that, in the United Kingdom, has resulted in a decrease in young audiences' exposure to products linked with childhood obesity.[413] Researchers in Australia have also documented that advertising healthy foods to children can increase positive attitudes toward the food and children's willingness to choose healthy food as a snack.[414]

RESEARCHERS

Many current studies of risky behaviors among adolescents, including drug use, sexual activity, and eating disorders, completely ignore the possibility of media influence.[132] Researchers need to incorporate measures of media use (and impact) into their studies of child and adolescent behavior. Longitudinal studies with children and adolescents representative of the population are needed to better understand the cumulative effect of media on the developing child and the differential effects of the media on distinct subpopulations of children.[411] As well, researchers need to stay abreast of evolving media technologies such as iPad "apps," both to document how they are used and by whom, as well as to determine their impact on the healthy development of children. With newer technology, researchers also specifically need to consider[415] the following:

1. The need for longitudinal research to examine the causal relationships between online participation and engaging in risk-related behaviors, such as aggression and sexual behaviors.
2. The major risk factors (ie, individual, environmental, social) that are related to a child or adolescent "acting" on this Internet exposure.

3. The need for specific research on children younger than 12, given their increasing use of the Internet. In particular, there is a strong need for studying those younger than 6 who have less capacity to "cope" with riskier online content.
4. Research on expanding platforms, such as mobile phones and virtual game environments, as well as peer-to-peer exchanges. Research on social networking sites is just now beginning to proliferate.
5. Increased research on public health issues, such as self-harm, suicide, drugs, and addiction.

GOVERNMENT

In the United States, Americans often experience a tension between 2 highly valued principles: protecting the free speech rights of media makers and advertisers and protecting the health and well-being of the nation's most vulnerable populations: children and adolescents. This has often meant that we regulate by "raised eyebrow"; that is, if Congress becomes concerned about particular content or practices, the industry offers to self-regulate. But the recent effort by the Working Group in Washington to rein in advertising of junk food and fast food shows that some industries are not even willing to engage in substantial self-regulation.[416] What is also lacking is often the follow-through needed to determine if a particular industry's self-regulatory practices are even effectively addressing the concerns.[292] For example, Coca-Cola has pledged to refrain from advertising to children; yet, the average child sees nearly 4 product placements of Coke on primetime TV every week.[417] Similarly, when regulations are "on the books," such as the Children's Television Act of 1990 (which mandates 3 hours per week of educational or informational programming for children on broadcast television networks), federal agencies do not rigorously enforce them.[418] With the explosion in digital media, it is time to revisit the roles of federal regulatory agencies, such as the Federal Communications Commission and the Federal Trade Commission.[419] It is critical for research experts and health care professionals to contribute to these deliberations.

Government could also provide more funding for media education efforts and for positive media content that encourages healthy lifestyles and choices (such as the Ready to Learn programs for preschoolers from the Department of Education). Through the National Institute of Mental Health, the government could also issue a new omnibus report to update current knowledge of media effects on children and adolescents and to stimulate new research efforts. The last such report was in 1982, well before the Internet, cell phones, and interactive advertising were even available. Amazingly, the government funds very little research on either traditional media or new media.

SUMMARY

During the past 50 years, thousands of research studies have revealed that the media can be a powerful teacher of children and adolescents and have a profound impact on their health. The media are not the leading cause of any major health problem in the United States, but they do contribute significantly to a variety of pediatric and adolescent health problems: aggressive behavior, sexual activity, drug use, obesity, sleep disorders, and others. Epidemiologically, the media contribute perhaps 10% to 20% to any specific health problem.[8,48,420] Given the sheer amount of time that children and teens spend with media (>7 hours a day), one would think that adult society would recognize the impact of media on young people's attitudes and behaviors. Sadly, many choose to ignore this potentially powerful influence. To date, too little has been done by parents, health care practitioners, schools, the entertainment industry, or the government to protect children and adolescents from harmful media effects and to maximize the powerfully prosocial aspects of modern media. More research is needed, but sufficient data exist to warrant both concern and increased action.

REFERENCES

1. Bushman BJ, Huesmann LR. Effects of televised violence on aggression. In: Singer DG, Singer JL, editors. Handbook of children and the media. Thousand Oaks (CA): Sage; 2001. p. 223–54.
2. Deveny K, Kelley R. Girls gone wild: what are celebs teaching kids? Newsweek 2007;40–7.
3. Ansen D. A handful of tangos in Paris. Newsweek 1999;66.
4. Eszterhas J. Hollywood's responsibility for smoking deaths. Available at: www.nytimes.com/2002/08/09/opinion/09ESZT.html. Accessed January 3, 2008.
5. Pipher M. Quoted in People Magazine. New York (NY): Time Warner Inc., June 3, 1996.
6. Boyer R, Levine D, Zensius N. TECHsex USA—youth sexuality and reproductive health in the digital age. Oakland (CA): ISIS, Inc.; 2011.
7. Boyd D. Why youth (heart) social network sites: the role of networked publics in teenage social life. In: Buckingham D, editor. MacArthur Foundation Series on Digital Learning—youth, identity, and digital media. Cambridge (MA): MIT Press; 2007. p. 119–42.
8. Strasburger VC, Wilson BJ, Jordan AB. Children, adolescents, and the media. 2nd edition. Thousand Oaks (CA): Sage; 2009.
9. Fisch S, Truglio R, Cole C. The impact of Sesame Street on preschool children: a review and synthesis of 30 years' of research. Media Psychol 1999;1:165–90.
10. Hogan MJ, Strasburger VC. Media and prosocial behavior in children and adolescents. In: Nucci L, Narvaez D, editors. Handbook of moral and character education. Mahwah (NJ): Lawrence Erlbaum; 2008. p. 537–53.
11. Mares M-L, Woodard EH. Effects of prosocial media content on children's social interactions. In: Singer DG, Singer JL, editors. Handbook of children and media. 2nd edition. Thousand Oaks (CA): Sage; 2012. p. 197–214.
12. Strasburger VC. Why do adolescent health researchers ignore the impact of the media? J Adolesc Health 2009;44:203–5.
13. Rideout V. Generation M2: Media in the lives of 8- to 18-year-olds. Menlo Park (CA): Kaiser Family Foundation; 2010.
14. Lenhart A. Teens and sexting. Washington, DC: Pew Internet & American Life Project; 2009. Available at: http://www.pewinternet.org/~/media//Files/Reports/2009/PIP_Teens_and_Sexting.pdf. Accessed June 27, 2011.
15. Jordan A, Bleakley A, Manganello J, et al. The role of television access in viewing time of US adolescents. J Child Media 2010;4(4):335–70.
16. Dennison BA, Erb TA, Jenkins PL. Television viewing and television in bedroom associated with overweight risk among low income preschool children. Pediatrics 2002;109(6):1028–35.
17. Jackson C, Brown JD, L'Engle KL. R-rated movies, bedroom televisions, and initiation of smoking by white and black adolescents. Arch Pediatr Adolesc Med 2007;161(3):260–8.
18. Garrison MM, Leikweg K, Christakis DA. Media use and child sleep: the impact of content, timing, and environment. Pediatrics 2011;128:29–35.

19. Rideout V, Roberts DF, Foehr UG. Generation M: Media in the lives of 8-18 year-olds. Menlo Park (CA): Kaiser Family Foundation; 2005.
20. Nielsen Company. Television, Internet and mobile usage in the U.S.: A2/M2 Three Screen Report. New York: Nielsen Company; 2009.
21. Rideout V, Lauricella A, Wartella E. Media use among white, black, Hispanic, and Asian American children. Evanston (IL): Northwestern University; 2011.
22. Rideout V. Zero to eight: children's media use in America. San Francisco: Common Sense Media; 2011. Available at: http://www.commonsensemedia.org/sites/default/files/research/zerotoeightfinal2011.pdf. Accessed December 3, 2011.
23. Nielsen Company. State of the media: TV usage trends: Q3 and Q4 2010. New York: Nielsen Company; 2011.
24. Lenhart A, Ling R, Campbell S, et al. Teens and mobile phones. Washington, DC: Pew Internet & American Life Project; 2010.
25. Vogel I, Vershuure H, van der Ploeg CP, et al. Adolescents and MP3 players: too many risks, too few precautions. Pediatrics 2009;123:e953–8.
26. Small G, Vorgan G. iBrain: surviving the technology alteration of the modern mind. New York: Harper Collins; 2008.
27. Lin L. Breadth-biased versus focused cognitive control in media multitasking behaviors. Proc Natl Acad Sci U S A 2009;106(37):15521–2.
28. Kohut A, Doherty C, Dimock M, et al. Internet gains on television as public's main news source. Washington, DC: Pew Research Center; 2011.
29. Hallin DC. Sound bite news: television coverage of elections, 1968-1988. J Commun 2006;42:5–24.
30. Robinson M. What sound bites are reported during the presidential campaign and why. 2007. Available at: http://www.asociatedcontent.com/article/252458/what_sound_bites_are_reported_during. Accessed June 29, 2011.
31. Bandura A. Social cognitive theory of mass communication. In: Bryant J, Oliver MB, editors. Media effects: advances in theory and research. 3rd edition. New York: Routledge; 2009. p. 94–124.
32. Huesmann LR. The role of social information processing and cognitive schema in the acquisition and maintenance of habitual aggressive behavior. In: Geen RG, Donnerstein E, editors. Human aggression: theories, research, and implications for policy. New York: Academic Press; 1998. p. 73–109.
33. Strasburger VC. Adolescents and the media: medical and psychological impact. Thousand Oaks (CA): Sage; 1995.
34. Brown JD, Halpern CT, L'Engle KL. Mass media as a sexual super peer for early maturing girls. J Adolesc Health 2005;36:420–7.
35. Hoffner C, Plotkin R, Buchanan M, et al. The third-person effect in perceptions of the influence of television violence. J Commun 2006;51(2):283–99.
36. Paul B, Salwen MB, Dupagne M. The third person effect: a meta-analysis of the perceptual hypothesis. In: Preiss R, Gayle B, Burrell N, et al, editors. Mass media effects research: advances through meta-analysis. Mahway (NJ): Lawrence Erlbaum; 2007. p. 81–102.
37. Strasburger VC, Council on Communications and Media. Media violence (policy statement). Pediatrics 2009;124:1495–503.
38. Smith A. Influence of TV crime programs on children's health. JAMA 1952;150:37.
39. Center on Media and Child Health. Available at: www.cmch.tv. Accessed July 25, 2011.
40. US Surgeon General's Scientific Advisory Committee on Television and Social Behavior. Television and growing up: the impact of televised violence: report

to the surgeon general. Rockville (MD): National Institute of Mental Health, US Public Health Service; 1972. Publication No. HSM 72-9090.

41. Pearl D, Bouthilet L, Lazar J. Television and behavior. Ten years of scientific progress and implications for the eighties. Rockville (MD): National Institute of Mental Health; 1982.

42. O'Toole ME. The school shooter: a threat assessment perspective. Quantico (VA): Federal Bureau of Investigation, US Department of Justice; 2000.

43. In the matter of violent television programming and its impact on children. Statement of Commissioner Deborah Taylor Tate. Federal Communications Commission; 2007. MB docket No. 04-261.

44. Gentile DA, Obert C, Sherwood NE, et al. Well-child exams in the video age: pediatricians and the American Academy of Pediatrics guidelines for children's media use. Pediatrics 2004;114(5):1235-41.

45. Strasburger VC. Go ahead punk, make my day: it's time for pediatricians to take action against media violence. Pediatrics 2007;119(6):e1398-9.

46. Murray JP. Media violence: the effects are both real and strong. Am Behav Sci 2008;51:1212-30.

47. Bushman BJ, Huesmann LR. Effects of violent media on aggression. In: Singer DG, Singer JL, editors. Handbook of children and the media. Los Angeles (CA): Sage; 2012. p. 231-48.

48. Comstock G, Strasburger VC. Media violence: Q&A. Adolesc Med 1993;4(3): 495-510.

49. Bushman BJ, Anderson CA. Comfortably numb: desensitizing effects of violent media on helping others. Psychol Sci 2009;20:273-7.

50. Ybarra ML, Diener-West M, Markow D, et al. Linkages between Internet and other media violence with seriously violent behavior by youth. Pediatrics 2008;122:929-37.

51. Cantor J. Mommy, I'm scared: how TV and movies frighten children and what we can do to protect them. New York: Harcourt Brace; 1998.

52. Federman J, editor. National television violence study, vol. 3. Thousand Oaks (CA): Sage; 1998.

53. Yokota F, Thompson KM. Violence in G-rated animated films. JAMA 2000; 283(20):2716-20.

54. Webb T, Jenkins L, Browne N, et al. Violent entertainment pitched to adolescents: an analysis of PG-13 films. Pediatrics 2007;119(6):e1219-29.

55. Worth KA, Chambers JG, Naussau DH, et al. Exposure of US adolescents to extremely violent movies. Pediatrics 2008;122:306-12.

56. Cheng TL, Brenner RA, Wright JL, et al. Children's violent television viewing: are parents monitoring? Pediatrics 2004;114(1):94-9.

57. Leone R, Barowski L. MPAA ratings creep: a longitudinal analysis of the PG-13 rating category in US movies. J Child Media 2011;5(1):53-69.

58. Herd DA. Changes in the prevalence of violent rap song lyrics 1979-1997. J Public Health Policy 2009;30(4):395-406.

59. Ybarra ML, Dierner-West M, Markow D, et al. Linkages between Internet and other media violence with seriously violent behavior by youth. Pediatrics 2008; 122(5):929-37.

60. Gentile DA. The rating systems for media products. In: Calvert S, Wilson B, editors. Handbook on children and media. Boston: Blackwell; 2007. p. 527-51.

61. Funk JB, Buchman DD. Playing violent video and computer games and adolescent self-concept. J Commun 1996;46(2):19-32.

62. Walsh D, Gentile DA, Walsh E, et al. Tenth annual mediawise video game report card. Minneapolis (MN): National Institute on Media and the Family; 2006. Available at: http://www.marketwire.com/press-release/10th-Annual-MediaWise-Video-Game-Report-Card-Console-Makers-Have-Evolved-Ratings-Have-671849.htm. Accessed July 27, 2011.

63. Anderson CA, Gentile DA, Dill KE. Prosocial, antisocial, and other effects of recreational video games. In: Singer DG, Singer JL, editors. Handbook of children and the media. 2nd edition. Los Angeles (CA): Sage; 2012. p. 249–72.

64. Wolak J, Mitchell KJ, Finkelhor D. Does online harassment constitute bullying? An exploration of online harassment by known peers and online-only contacts. J Adolesc Health 2007;41:S51–8.

65. Ybarra ML, Diener-West M, Leaf PJ. Examining the overlap in Internet harassment and school bullying: implications for school intervention. J Adolesc Health 2007;41:S42–50.

66. Kowalski RM, Limber SP. Electronic bullying among middle school students. J Adolesc Health 2007;41:S22–30.

67. Hertz MF, David-Perdon C. Electronic media and youth violence: a CDC issue brief for educators and caregivers. Atlanta (GA): Centers for Disease Control; 2008.

68. Tokunaga RS. Following you home from school: a critical review and synthesis of research on cyberbullying victimization. Comput Human Behav 2010;26:277–87.

69. Ybarra ML, Mitchell KJ, Korchmaros JD. National trends in exposure to and experiences of violence on the Internet among children. Pediatrics 2011;128: e1376–86.

70. Williams KR, Guerra NG. Prevalence and predictors of Internet bullying. J Adolesc Health 2007;S14–21.

71. Ybarra ML, Espelage DL, Mitchell KJ. The co-occurrence of Internet harassment and unwanted sexual solicitation victimization and perpetration: associations with psychosocial indicators. J Adolesc Health 2007;S31–41.

72. McIntosh WD, Murray JD, Murray RM, et al. What's so funny about a poke in the eye? The prevalence of violence in comedy films and its relation to social and economic threat in the United States, 1951-2000. Mass Comm Soc 2003;6:345–60.

73. Kirsh SJ. Children, adolescents, and media violence: a critical look at the research. 2nd edition. Thousand Oaks (CA): Sage; 2012.

74. Anderson CA, Berkowitz L, Donnerstein E, et al. The influence of media violence on youth. Psychol Sci Public Interest 2003;4(3):81–110.

75. Boxer P, Huesmann LR, Bushman BJ, et al. The role of violent media preference in cumulative developmental risk for violence and general aggression. J Youth Adolesc 2009;38:417–28.

76. Donnerstein E. The Internet. In: Strasburger VC, Wilson BJ, Jordan AB. Children, adolescents, and the media. 3rd edition. Thousand Oaks (CA): Sage; 2013, in press.

77. Strasburger VC, Grossman D. How many more Columbines? What can pediatricians do about school and media violence? Pediatr Ann 2001;30:87–94.

78. Bleakley A, Hennessy M, Fishbein M, et al. How sources of sexual information relate to adolescents' beliefs about sex. Am J Health Behav 2009;33(1):37–48.

79. Strasburger VC. Adolescents, sex, and the media. Pediatr Clin North Am 2012; 23(1):15–33.

80. Strasburger VC, Council on Communications and Media. Sexuality, contraception, and the media (policy statement). Pediatrics 2010;126:576–82.

81. Brown JD, Strasburger VC. From Calvin Klein to Paris Hilton and MySpace: adolescents, sex, and the media. Adolesc Med State Art Rev 2007;18:484–507.

82. Wright PJ. Mass media effects on youth sexual behavior: assessing the claim for causality. Comm Yearbk 2011;35:343–86.

83. National Campaign to Prevent Teen and Unplanned Pregnancy. Teen child-bearing in the United States, final 2008 birth data. Washington, DC: NCPTUP; 2010.

84. Centers for Disease Control and Prevention. Vital signs: teen pregnancy—United States, 1991-2009. MMWR Morb Mortal Wkly Rep 2011;60(13): 414–20.

85. Centers for Disease Control and Prevention. Youth risk behavior surveillance—United States, 2009. MMWR Morb Mortal Wkly Rep 2010;59(No. SS-5):1–142.

86. Kunkel D, Eyal K, Finnerty K, et al. Sex on TV 4: a biennial report to the Kaiser Family Foundation. Menlo Park (CA): Kaiser Family Foundation; 2005.

87. Ybarra M. Digital adolescence: myths and truths about growing up with technology. Presented at annual meeting of American Psychological Association. Washington, DC: August 6, 2011.

88. Kunkel D, Eyal K, Donnerstein E, et al. Sexual socialization messages on entertainment television: comparing content trends 1997-2002. Media Psychol 2007; 9:595–622.

89. Zurbriggen EL, Morgan EM. Who wants to marry a millionaire? Reality dating television programs, attitudes towards sex, and sexual behaviors. Sex Roles 2006;54:1–17.

90. Tomashoff C. Are the kids all right? TV Guide 2011;12–4.

91. Parents Television Council. Sexualized teen girls: tinseltown's new target. Washington, DC: Parents Television Council; 2010.

92. Williams ME. Television's season of the vagina. 2011. Available at: http://www.salon.com/2011/09/26/vagina_sitcom_season/. Accessed December 2, 2011.

93. Carter B. This year's hot TV trend is anatomically correct. NY Times 2011. Available at: http://www.nytimes.com/2011/09/22/arts/television/this-years-hot-tv-trend-is-a-word.html?pagewanted=all. Accessed December 2, 2011.

94. Tuck L. Viewer discretion advised. POZ. com. Available at: http://www.poz.com/articles/Teens_HIV_TV_2557_19656.shtml. Accessed August 22, 2011.

95. Bashir M. Porn in hi-definition: too much detail? ABC News.com; 2007. Available at: http://abcnews.go.com/Nightline/story?id=2854981&page=1. Accessed July 28, 2011.

96. Wingood GM, DiClemente RJ, Harrington K, et al. Exposure to X-rated movies and adolescents' sexual and contraceptive-related attitudes and behaviors. Pediatrics 2001;107:1116–9.

97. Wright PJ, Malamuth NM, Donnerstein E. Research on sex in the media: what do we know about effects on children and adolescents? In: Singer DG, Singer JL, editors. Handbook of children and the media. 2nd edition. Los Angeles (CA): Sage; 2012. p. 273–302.

98. Bridges AJ, Wosnitzer R, Scharrer E, et al. Aggression and sexual behavior in best-selling pornography videos: a content analysis update. Violence Against Women 2010;16(10):1065–85.

99. Primack BA, Gold MA, Schwarz EB, et al. Degrading and non-degrading sex in popular music: a content analysis. Public Health Rep 2008;123:593–600.

100. Hall PC, West JH, Hill S. Sexualization in lyrics of popular music from 1959 to 2009: implications for sexuality educators. Sexuality and Culture 2011. DOI: 10.1007/s12119-011-9103-4.

101. Walsh-Childers K, Gotthoffer A, Lepre CR. From "just the facts" to "downright salacious": teens' and women's magazines' coverage of sex and sexual health. In: Brown JD, Steele JR, Walsh-Childers K, editors. Sexual teens, sexual media. Hillsdale (NJ): Lawrence Erlbaum; 2002. p. 153–71.

102. Reichert T, Carpenter C. An update on sex in magazine advertising: 1983 to 2003. Journal Mass Commun Q 2004;81:823–37.

103. Wingood GM, DiClemente RJ, Bernhardt JM, et al. A prospective study of exposure to rap music videos and African American female adolescents' health. Am J Public Health 2003;93:437–9.

104. Collins RL, Elliott MN, Berry SH, et al. Watching sex on television predicts adolescent initiation of sexual behavior. Pediatrics 2004;114:e280–9.

105. Ashby SL, Arcari CM, Edmonson MB. Television viewing and risk of sexual initiation by young adolescents. Arch Pediatr Adolesc Med 2006;160:375–80.

106. Brown JD, L'Engle K, Pardun CJ, et al. Sexy media matter: exposure to sexual content in music, movies, television, and magazines predicts black and white adolescents' sexual behavior. Pediatrics 2006;117:1018–27.

107. Martino SC, Collins RL, Elliott MN, et al. Exposure to degrading versus nondegrading music lyrics and sexual behavior among youth. Pediatrics 2006;118: e430–41.

108. Chandra A, Martino SC, Collins RL, et al. Does watching sex on television predict teen pregnancy? Findings from a National Longitudinal Survey of Youth. Pediatrics 2008;122:1047–54.

109. Bersamin M, Todd M, Fisher DA, et al. Parenting practices and adolescent sexual behavior: a longitudinal study. J Marriage Fam 2008;70:97–112.

110. Bleakley A, Hennessy M, Fishbein M, et al. It works both ways: The relationship between exposure to sexual content in the media and adolescent sexual behavior. Media Psychol 2008;11:443–61.

111. Peter J, Valkenburg PM. Adolescents' exposure to sexually explicit Internet material and sexual preoccupancy: a three-wave panel study. Media Psychol 2008;11:207–34.

112. Brown JD, L'Engle KL. X-rated: sexual attitudes and behaviors associated with U.S. early adolescents' exposure to sexually explicit media. Communic Res 2009;36:129–51.

113. Delgado H, Austin SB, Rich M, et al. Exposure to adult-targeted television and movies during childhood increases risk of initiation of early intercourse [abstract]. Presented at Pediatric Academic Societies meeting. Baltimore, May 4, 2009.

114. Hennessy M, Bleakley A, Fishbein M, et al. Estimating the longitudinal association between adolescent sexual behavior and exposure to sexual media content. J Sex Res 2009;46:1–11.

115. Bersamin MM, Bourdeau B, Fisher DA, et al. Television use, sexual behavior, and relationship status at last oral sex and vaginal intercourse. Sexuality and Culture 2010;14:157–68.

116. Ybarra ML, Mitchell KJ, Hamburger M, et al. X-rated material and perpetration of sexually aggressive behavior among children and adolescents: is there a link? Aggress Behav 2011;37:1–18.

117. Martino SC, Collins RL, Kanouse DE, et al. Social cognitive processes mediating the relationship between exposure to television's sexual content and adolescents' sexual behavior. J Pers Soc Psychol 2005;89:914–24.

118. L'Engle KL, Jackson C. Socialization influences on early adolescents' cognitive susceptibility and transition to sexual intercourse. J Res Adolesc 2008;18:353–78.

119. Gottfried JA, Vaala SE, Bleakley A, et al. Does the effect of exposure to TV sex on adolescent sexual behavior vary by genre? Communic Res 2011. Available at: http://crx.sagepub.com/content/early/2011/07/16/0093650211415399.full. pdf+html. Accessed March 16, 2012.

120. Primack BA, Douglas EL, Fine MJ, et al. Exposure to sexual lyrics and sexual experience among urban adolescents. Am J Prev Med 2009;36:317–23.

121. Newman AA. Pigs with cellphones, but no condoms. New York Times 2007;B1. Available at: http://www.nytimes.com/2007/06/18/business/media/18adcol.html? adxnnl=1&adxnnlx=1313772936–1WXEee4fVg80ZPLh1fojeA. Accessed August 19, 2011.

122. Brodesser-akner C. Sex on TV is ok as long as it's not safe. Advert Age 2007. Available at: http://adage.com/article/news/sex-tv-long-safe/120489/. Accessed December 3, 2011.

123. Snowbeck C. FDA tells Levitra to cool it with ad. Post-Gazette 2005. Available at: www.post-gazette.com/pg/05109/490334-28.stm. Accessed August 22, 2011.

124. Campbell S. Promotional spending for prescription drugs. Washington, DC: Congressional Budget Office; 2009. Available at: http://www.cbo.gov/ftpdocs/ 105xx/doc10522/12-02-DrugPromo_Brief.pdf. Accessed August 22, 2011.

125. Wolk LI, Rosenbaum R. The benefits of school-based condom availability: cross-sectional analysis of a comprehensive high school-based program. J Adolesc Health 1995;17:184–8.

126. Furstenberg FF Jr, Geitz LM, Teitler JO, et al. Does condom availability make a difference? An evaluation of Philadelphia's health resource centers. Fam Plann Perspect 1997;29:123–7.

127. Guttmacher S, Lieberman L, Ward D, et al. Condom availability in New York City public high schools: relationships to condom use and sexual behavior. Am J Public Health 1997;87:1427–33.

128. Jemmott JB III, Jemmott LS, Fong GT. Abstinence and safer sex: HIV risk-reduction interventions for African American adolescents. JAMA 1998;279:1529–36.

129. Schuster MA, Bell RM, Berry SH, et al. Impact of a high-school condom availability program on sexual attitudes and behaviors. Fam Plann Perspect 1998; 30:67–72.

130. Kirby D, Brener ND, Brown NL, et al. The impact of condom distribution in Seattle schools on sexual behavior and condom use. Am J Public Health 1999;89:182–7.

131. Blake SM, Ledsky R, Goodenow C, et al. Condom availability programs in Massachusetts high schools: relationships with condom use and sexual behavior. Am J Public Health 2003;93:955–62.

132. Sellers DE, McGraw SA, McKinlay JB. Does the promotion and distribution of condoms increase sexual activity? Evidence from an HIV prevention program for Latino youth. Am J Public Health 1994;84:1952–9.

133. Wretzel SR, Visintainer PF, Koenigs LMP. Condom availability program in an inner city public school: effect on the rates of gonorrhea and chlamydia infection. J Adolesc Health 2011;49(3):324–6.

134. Kristof N. Beyond chastity belts. New York Times 2006;A25. Available at: http:// select.nytimes.com/2006/05/02/opinion/02kristof.html?_r=2. Accessed August 22, 2011. 131.

135. Rideout V. Generation RX.Com: how young people use the Internet for health information. Menlo Park (CA): Kaiser Family Foundation; 2001.

136. Wolak J, Mitchell K, Finkelhor D. Unwanted and wanted exposure to online pornography in a national sample of youth Internet users. Pediatrics 2007; 119:247–57.

137. Sabina C, Wolak J, Finkelhor D. The nature and dynamics of Internet pornography exposure for youth. Cyberpsychol Behav 2008;11:1–3.
138. Moyer MW. The sunny side of smut. Sci Am 2011;14–5.
139. Braun-Courville DK, Rojas M. Exposure to sexually explicit web sites and adolescent sexual attitudes and behaviors. J Adolesc Health 2009;45:156–62.
140. Lounsbury K, Mitchell KJ, Finkelhor D. The true prevalence of "sexting." Durham (NH): Crimes Against Children Research Center, University of New Hampshire; 2011.
141. National Campaign to Prevent Teen and Unplanned Pregnancy. Sex and tech. Washington, DC: National Campaign to Prevent Teen and Unplanned Pregnancy; 2008.
142. Cox Communications. Teen Online & Wireless Safety Survey: cyberbullying, sexting, and parental controls. Atlanta (GA): Cox Communications; 2009.
143. Associated Press and MTV. AP-MTV Digital Abuse Study, executive summary. Available at: http://www.athinline.org/MTV-AP_Digital_Abuse_Study_Executive_Summary.pdf. Accessed August 17, 2011.
144. Phippen A. Sharing personal images and videos among young people. South West Grid for Learning & University of Plymouth, UK. Available at: http://www.swgfl.org.uk/Staying-Safe/Files/Documents/sexting-summary. Accessed August 17, 2011.
145. Mitchell K, Finkelhor D, Jones L, et al. Prevalence and characteristics of youth sexting: a national study. Pediatrics 2012;129:1–8.
146. Calvert C. Sex, cell phones, privacy, and the first amendment: when children become child pornographers and the Lolita Effect undermines the law. Comm-Law Conspectus 2009;18:1–65.
147. Klepper D. Teen sexting penalties may be relaxed by states. The Huffington Post 2011. Available at: http://www.huffingtonpost.com/2011/06/13/teen-sexting-penalties_n_875783.html?view=print. Accessed August 17, 2011.
148. Wolak J, Finkelhor D, Mitchell KJ. How often are teens arrested for sexting? Data from a national sample of police cases. Pediatrics 2012;129:1–9.
149. Lithwick D. Textual misconduct. Slate, 2009. Available at: http://www.slate.com/id/2211169/. Accessed August 22, 2011.
150. Wilson C. Feds: online "sextortion" of teens on the rise. Associated Press; 2010. Available at: http://www.msnbc.msn.com/id/38714259/ns/technology_and_science-security/t/feds-online-sextortion-teens-rise/. Accessed August 22, 2011.
151. Moreno MA, Parks MR, Zimmerman FJ, et al. Display of health risk behavior on MySpace by adolescents. Arch Pediatr Adolesc Med 2009;163:27–34.
152. Moreno MA, Brockman L, Rogers CB, et al. An evaluation of the distribution of sexual references among "top 8" MySpace friends. J Adolesc Health 2010;47(4):418–20.
153. Joshi M. Social sites may provide clues to teens' sexual intentions. Health News 2010. Available at: http://www.topnews.in/health/social-sites-may-provide-clues-teens-sexual-intentions-27065. Accessed April 4, 2012.
154. Mitchell KJ, Wolak J, Finkelhor D. Trends in youth reports of sexual solicitations, harassment, and unwanted exposure to pornography on the Internet. J Adolesc Health 2007;40:116–26.
155. Ybarra ML, Mitchell KH. How risky are social networking sites? A comparison of places online where youth sexual solicitation and harassment occurs. Pediatrics 2008;121(2):e350–7.
156. Mitchell KJ, Finkelhor D, Jones LM, et al. Use of social networking sites in online sex crimes against minors: an examination of national incidence and means of utilization. J Adolesc Health 2010;47:183–90.

157. Noll JG, Shenk CE, Barnes JE, et al. Childhood abuse, avatar choices, and other risk factors associated with Internet-initiated victimization of adolescent girls. Pediatrics 2009;123:e1078–83.

158. Wolak J, Finkelhor D, Mitchell KH, et al. Online "predators" and their victims: myths, realities, and implications for prevention and treatment. Am Psychol 2008;63:111–28.

159. Brodie M, Foehr U, Rideout V, et al. Communicating health information through the entertainment media. Health Aff (Millwood) 2001;20(1):192–9.

160. Collins RL, Elliott MN, Berry SH, et al. Entertainment television as a healthy sex educator: the impact of condom-efficacy information in an episode of Friends. Pediatrics 2003;112(5):1115–21.

161. Rideout V. Television as a health educator: a case study of Grey's Anatomy. Menlo Park (CA): Kaiser Family Foundation; 2008.

162. Armstrong J. Gay teens on TV. TV Guide 2011;34–41.

163. Hoffman J. Fighting teenage pregnancy with MTV stars as Exhibit A. New York Times 2011;1–11.

164. National Campaign to Prevent Teen and Unplanned Pregnancy. Is media glamorizing teen pregnancy [press release]. Washington, DC: NCPTUP; 2010.

165. Pinkleton BE, Austin EW, Cohen M, et al. Effects of a peer-led media literacy curriculum on adolescents' knowledge and attitudes toward sexual behavior and media portrayals of sex. Health Commun 2008;23(5):462–72.

166. DuRant RH, Wolfson M, LaFrance B, et al. An evaluation of a mass media campaign to encourage parents of adolescents to talk to their children about sex. J Adolesc Health 2006;38(3):298,e1–9.

167. Collins RL, Martino SC, Shaw R. Influence of new media on adolescent sexual health: evidence and opportunities. Santa Monica (CA): RAND; 2011.

168. Levine D, McCright J, Dobkin L, et al. SEXINFO: a sexual health text messaging service for San Francisco youth. Am J Public Health 2008;98:393–5.

169. Winston L. Good, better, best: school-based STD screening in Washington, DC. Washington, DC: U.S. Department of Health; 2010.

170. Paperny DM, Starn JR. Adolescent pregnancy prevention by health education computer games: computer-assisted instruction of knowledge and attitudes. Pediatrics 1989;83:742–52.

171. Tortolero SR, Markham CM, Peskin MF, et al. It's your game: keep it real: delaying sexual behavior with an effective middle school program. J Adolesc Health 2009;46:169–79.

172. Freimuth VS, Snyder L, Nadorff GG, et al. Assessing the viral transmission of HIV mobile media messages. Paper presented at CDC Annual Conference on Health Communication, Marketing, and Media. Atlanta, August 12, 2009.

173. Moreno MA, VanderStoep A, Parks MR, et al. Reducing at-risk adolescents' display of risk behavior on a social networking web site. Arch Pediatr Adolesc Med 2009;163:35–41.

174. Strasburger VC, Council on Communications and Media. Children, adolescents, substance abuse, and the media. Pediatrics 2010;126:791–9.

175. Strasburger VC. Children, adolescents, drugs, and the media. In: Singer DG, Singer JL, editors. Handbook children and the media. 2nd edition. Los Angeles (CA): Sage; 2012. p. 419–54.

176. American Academy of Pediatrics. Committee on Substance Abuse. Tobacco use: a pediatric disease. Pediatrics 2009;124(5):1474–87.

177. Johnston LD, O'Malley PM, Bachman JG, et al. Monitoring the future national results on adolescent drug use: overview of key findings, 2010. Ann Arbor (MI): Institute for Social Research, University of Michigan; 2011.

178. US Department of Health and Human Services. The Surgeon General's call to action to prevent and reduce underage drinking. Rockville (MD): US Department of Health and Human Services; 2007.

179. Federal Trade Commission. Federal Trade Commission cigarette report for 2007 and 2008. Washington, DC: FTC; 2011. Available at: http://www.ftc.gov/os/2011/07/110729cigarettereport.pdf. Accessed August 27, 2011.

180. Fritschler AL, Hoefler JM. Smoking & politics: policy making and the federal bureaucracy. 6th edition. Upper Saddle River (NJ): Prentice Hall; 2006.

181. US Department of Health and Human Services. Preventing tobacco use among young people: report of the Surgeon General. Washington, DC: US Government Printing Office; 1994.

182. Pierce JP, Messer K, James LE, et al. Camel No. 9 cigarette-marketing campaign targeted young girls. Pediatrics 2010;125:619–26.

183. Wellman RJ, Sugarman DB, DiFranza J, et al. The extent to which tobacco marketing and tobacco use in films contribute to children's use of tobacco. Arch Pediatr Adolesc Med 2006;160(12):1285–96.

184. Centers for Disease Control. Cigarette brand preference among middle and high school students who are established smokers—United States, 2004 and 2006. MMWR Morb Mortal Wkly Rep 2009;58:112–5.

185. Cortese DK, Lewis MJ, Ling PM. Tobacco industry lifestyle magazines targeted to young adults. J Adolesc Health Care 2009;45:268–80.

186. DiFranza JR, Wellman RJ, Sargent JD, et al. Tobacco Consortium, Center for Child Health Research of the American Academy of Pediatrics. Tobacco promotion and the initiation of tobacco use: assessing the evidence for causality. Pediatrics 2006;117(6):e1237–48.

187. Sargent J, Gibson J, Heatherton T. Comparing the effects of entertainment media and tobacco marketing on youth smoking. Tob Control 2009;18(1): 47–53.

188. Hanewinkel R, Isensee B, Sargent JD, et al. Cigarette advertising and teen smoking initiation. Pediatrics 2011;127:e271–8.

189. US Food and Drug Administration. Overview: Cigarette health warnings. Available at: http://www.fda.gov/TobaccoProducts/Labeling/ucm259214.htm#High_Resolution_Image_Formats. Accessed March 16, 2012.

190. Center on Alcohol Marketing and Youth. Alcohol advertising and youth [fact sheet]. Washington, DC: Center on Alcohol Marketing and Youth; 2007.

191. Grube JW, Waiters E. Alcohol in the media: content and effects on drinking beliefs and behaviors among youth. Adolesc Med Clin 2005;16(2):327–43.

192. Jernigan DH. Importance of reducing youth exposure to alcohol advertising. Arch Pediatr Adolesc Med 2006;160(1):100–2.

193. Center on Alcohol Marketing and Youth. Youth exposure to alcohol advertising on television, 2001-2009. Baltimore (MD): CAMY; 2010.

194. Tanski SE, McClure AC, Jernigan DH, et al. Alcohol brand preference and binge drinking among adolescents. Arch Pediatr Adolesc Med 2011;165:675–6.

195. Center on Alcohol Marketing and Youth. Youth exposure to alcohol advertising in national magazines, 2001-2008. Baltimore (MD): CAMY; 2010.

196. Henriksen L, Feighery EC, Schleicher NC, et al. Receptivity to alcohol marketing predicts initiation of alcohol use. J Adolesc Health 2009;42:28–35.

197. Anderson P, de Bruijn A, Angus K, et al. Impact of alcohol advertising and media exposure on adolescent alcohol use: a systematic review of longitudinal studies. Alcohol Alcohol 2009;44:229–43.

198. McClure AC, Stoolmiller M, Tanski SE, et al. Alcohol-branded merchandise and its association with drinking attitudes and outcomes in US adolescents. Arch Pediatr Adolesc Med 2009;163:211–7.

199. Smith LA, Foxcroft DR. The effect of alcohol advertising, marketing and portrayal on drinking behavior in young people: systematic review of prospective cohort studies. BMC Public Health 2009;9:51. Available at: http://www.biomedcentral.com/1471-2458/9/51. Accessed March 16, 2012.

200. Jernigan DH. Alcohol-branded merchandise. Arch Pediatr Adolesc Med 2009; 163(3):278–9.

201. Morgenstern M, Isensee B, Sargent JD, et al. Attitudes as mediators of the longitudinal association between alcohol advertising and youth drinking. Arch Pediatr Adolesc Med 2011;165:610–6.

202. Stange KC. Time to ban direct-to-consumer prescription drug marketing. Ann Fam Med 2007;5:101–4.

203. Rubin A. Prescription drugs and the cost of advertising them. 2007. Available at: www.therubins.com/geninfo/advertise2.htm. Accessed August 28, 2011.

204. Angell M. The truth about the drug companies: how they deceive us and what to do about it. New York: Random House; 2005.

205. American Legacy Foundation. Trends in top box-office movie tobacco use: 1996 –2004. Washington, DC: American Legacy Foundation; 2006.

206. Sargent JD, Tanski SE, Gibson J. Exposure to movie smoking among US adolescents aged 10 to 14 years: a population estimate. Pediatrics 2007;119(5): e1167–76.

207. Goldstein AO, Sobel RA, Newman GR. Tobacco and alcohol use in G-rated children's animated films. JAMA 1999;281(12):1131–6.

208. Sargent JD, Heatherton TF. Comparison of trends for adolescent smoking and smoking in movies, 1990–2007. JAMA 2009;301(21):2211–3.

209. Glantz SA, Titus K, Mitchell S, et al. Smoking in top-grossing movies—United States, 1991–2009. MMWR Morb Mortal Wkly Rep 2010;59(32):1014–7.

210. Dalton MA, Sargent JD, Beach ML, et al. Effect of viewing smoking in movies on adolescent smoking initiation: a cohort study. Lancet 2003;362(9380):281–5.

211. Sargent JD, Beach ML, Adachi-Mejia AM, et al. Exposure to movie smoking: its relation to smoking initiation among US adolescents. Pediatrics 2005;116:1183–91.

212. National Cancer Institute. The role of the media in promoting and reducing tobacco use. Tobacco Control Monograph No. 19. Bethesda (MD): U.S. Department of Health and Human Services, National Institutes of Health, National Cancer Institute; 2008. NIH Pub. No. 07–6242.

213. Titus-Ernstoff L, Dalton MA, Adachi-Mejia AM, et al. Longitudinal study of viewing smoking in movies and initiation of smoking by children. Pediatrics 2008;121(1):15–21.

214. Dalton M, Beach M, Adachi-Mejia AM, et al. Early exposure to movie smoking predicts established smoking by older teens and young adults. Pediatrics 2009;123:e551–8.

215. Heatherton TF, Sargent JD. Does watching smoking in movies promote teenage smoking? Curr Dir Psychol Sci 2009;18:63–7.

216. Tanski SE, Stoolmiller M, Dal Cin S, et al. Movie characters smoking and adolescent smoking: who matters more, good guys or bad guys? Pediatrics 2009;124: 135–43.

217. Morgenstern M, Poelen EAP, Sholte R, et al. Smoking in movies and adolescent smoking: cross- cultural study in six European countries. Thorax 2011. Published online August 25, 2011. Available at: http://thorax.bmj.com/content/early/2011/08/25/thoraxjnl-2011-200489.short? Accessed August 30, 2011.

218. Dalton MA, Adachi-Meija AM, Longacre MR, et al. Parental rules and monitoring of children's movie viewing associated with children's risk for smoking and drinking. Pediatrics 2006;118(5):1932–42.

219. Jago R, Davison KK, Thompson J, et al. Parental sedentary restriction, maternal parenting style, and television viewing among 10- to 11-year-olds. Pediatrics 2011;128(3):e572–8.

220. Cullen J, Sokol NA, Slawek D, et al. Depictions of tobacco use in 2007 broadcast television programming popular among US youth. Arch Pediatr Adolesc Med 2011;165:147–51.

221. Healton CG, Watson-Stryker ES, Allen JA, et al. Televised movie trailers: undermining restrictions on advertising tobacco to youth. Arch Pediatr Adolesc Med 2006;160:885–8.

222. Hanewinkel R. Cigarette smoking and perception of a movie character in a film trailer. Arch Pediatr Adolesc Med 2009;163:15–8.

223. Murphy ST. How healthy is prime time? An analysis of health content in popular prime time television programs. Menlo Park (CA): Kaiser Family Foundation; 2008.

224. Gruber EL, Thau HM, Hill DL, et al. Alcohol, tobacco and illicit substances in music videos: a content analysis of prevalence and genre. J Adolesc Health 2005;37(1):81–3.

225. National Center on Addiction and Substance Abuse. National survey of American attitudes on substance abuse XVI: teens and parents. New York: Columbia University; 2011. Available at: http://www.casacolumbia.org/upload/2011/20110824teensurveyreport.pdf. Accessed August 28, 2011.

226. Sargent JD, Wills TA, Stoolmiller M, et al. Alcohol use in motion pictures and its relation to early-onset teen drinking. J Stud Alcohol 2006;67:54–65.

227. Primack BA, Kraemer KL, Fine MJ, et al. Media exposure and marijuana and alcohol use among adolescents. Subst Use Misuse 2009;44(5):722–39.

228. Wills TA, Sargent JD, Gibbons FX, et al. Movie exposure to alcohol cues and adolescent alcohol problems: a longitudinal analysis in a national sample. Psychol Addict Behav 2009;23(1):23–5.

229. Hanewinkel R, Sargent JD. Longitudinal study of exposure to entertainment media and alcohol use among German adolescents. Pediatrics 2009;123:989–95.

230. National Center on Addiction and Substance Abuse. National survey of American attitudes on substance abuse IX: teens and parents. New York: National Center on Addiction and Substance Abuse; 2005.

231. Dalton MA, Bernhardt AM, Gibson JJ, et al. Use of cigarettes and alcohol by preschoolers while role-playing as adults. Arch Pediatr Adolesc Med 2005;159(9):854–9.

232. Engels RC, Hermans R, van Baaren RB, et al. Alcohol portrayal on television affects actual drinking behaviour. Alcohol Alcohol 2009;44(3):244–9.

233. Callister M, Coyne SM, Robinson T, et al. "Three sheets to the wind": substance use in teen-centered film from 1980 to 2007. Addiction Res Theor 2011. DOI: 10.3109/16066359.2011.552818. Published online on May 23, 2011.

234. Christenson PG, Henriksen L, Roberts DF. Substance use in popular prime-time television. Washington, DC: Office of National Drug Policy Control; 2000.

235. Halperin S. Going to pot. Entertainment Weekly 2008;38–41.

236. Primack BA, Douglas EL, Kraemer KL. Exposure to cannabis in popular music and cannabis use among adolescents. Addiction 2010;105(3):515–23.

237. Jenssen BP, Klein JD, Salazar LR, et al. Exposure to tobacco on the Internet: content analysis of adolescents' Internet use. Pediatrics 2009;124:e180–6.

238. Moreno MA, Briner LR, Williams A, et al. A content analysis of displayed alcohol references on a social networking web site. J Adolesc Health 2010; 47:168–72.

239. Moreno MA, Briner LR, Williams A, et al. Real use or "real cool": adolescents speak out about displayed alcohol references on social networking websites. J Adolesc Health 2009;45:420–2.

240. Hitti M. Teens buying alcohol online. WebMD Medical News 2006. Available at: http://www.webmd.com/parenting/news/20060811/teens-buy-alcohol-online. Accessed August 28, 2011.

241. C.S. Mott Children's Hospital. National poll on children's health. Vol. 13, No. 3. August 15, 2011. Available at: http://www.med.umich.edu/mott/npch/pdf/081511toptenreport.pdf. Accessed September 1, 2011.

242. Special Feature. Obesity rates spin out of control. Nutrition Action HealthLetter 2011;11.

243. Ogden C, Carroll M. Prevalence of obesity among children and adolescents: United States, trends 1963-1965 through 2007-2008. Available at: http://www.cdc.gov/nchs/data/hestat/obesity_child_07_08/obesity_child_07_08.pdf. Accessed August 29, 2011.

244. Balkau B, Deanfield JE, Despres J-P, et al. International day for the evaluation of abdominal obesity (IDEA). A study of waist circumference, cardiovascular disease, and diabetes mellitus in 168,000 primary care patients in 63 countries. Circulation 2007;116:1942–51.

245. Danaei G, Finucane MM, Lu Y, et al. National, regional, and global trends in fasting plasma glucose and diabetes prevalence since 1980: systematic analysis of health examination surveys and epidemiological studies with 370 country-years and 2.7 million participants. Lancet 2011;378:31–40.

246. Today USA. Obesity costs U.S. $168 billion, study finds. 2010. Available at: http://www.usatoday.com/yourlife/fitness/2010-10-18-obesity-costs_N.htm. Accessed August 29, 2011.

247. Jordan A. Children's television viewing and childhood obesity. Pediatr Ann 2010; 39(9):569–73.

248. Dennison BA, Edmunds LS. The role of television in childhood obesity. Progr Pediatr Cardiol 2008;25(2):191–7.

249. Hancox RJ, Milne BJ, Poulton R. Association between child and adolescent television viewing and adult health: a longitudinal birth cohort study. Lancet 2004; 364(9430):257–62.

250. Viner RM, Cole TJ. Television viewing in early childhood predicts adult body mass index. J Pediatr 2005;147(4):429–35.

251. Reilly JJ, Armstrong J, Dorosty AR, et al. Early life risk factors for obesity in childhood: cohort study. BMJ 2005;330(7504):1357.

252. Sugimori H, Yoshida K, Izuno T, et al. Analysis of factors that influence body mass index from ages 3 to 6 years: a study based on the Toyama cohort study. Pediatr Int 2004;46(3):302–10.

253. Proctor MH, Moore LL, Gao D, et al. Television viewing and change in body fat from preschool to early adolescence: the Framingham Children's Study. Int J Obes Relat Metab Disord 2003;27:827–33.

254. Henderson VR. Longitudinal associations between television viewing and body mass index among white and black girls. J Adolesc Health 2007;41:544–50.

255. Mendoza JA, Zimmerman FJ, Christakis DA. Television viewing, computer use, obesity, and adiposity in US preschool children. Int J Behav Nutr Phys Act 2007;4:44. Available at: http://www.ijbnpa.org/content/4/1/44. Accessed August 31, 2011.

256. Sisson SB, Broyles ST, Baker BL, et al. Screen time, physical activity, and overweight in U.S. youth: National Survey of Children's Health 2003. J Adolesc Health 2010;47:309–11.

257. Zimmerman FJ, Bell JF. Associations of television content type and obesity in children. Am J Public Health 2010;100:334–40.

258. Anderson SE, Whitaker RC. Household routines and obesity in US preschool-age children. Pediatrics 2010;125:420–8.

259. Hoelscher PA, Springer AE, Brown HS, et al. Physical activity, watching television, and the risk of obesity in students, Texas, 2004-2006. Prev Chronic Dis 2011;8(3). Available at: http://www.cdc.gov/pcd/issues/2011/may/10_0007.htm. Accessed August 31, 2011.

260. Salmon J, Campbell KJ, Crawford DA. Television viewing habits associated with obesity risk factors: a survey of Melbourne schoolchildren. Med J Aust 2006;184:64–7.

261. Iannotti RJ, Kogan MD, Janssen I, et al. Patterns of adolescent physical activity, screen-based media use, and positive and negative health indicators in the U.S. and Canada. J Adolesc Health 2009;44:493–9.

262. Jackson DM, Djafarian K, Stewart J, et al. Increased television viewing is associated with elevated body fatness but not with lower total energy expenditure in children. Am J Clin Nutr 2009;89:1031–6.

263. Ozmert EN, Ozdemir R, Pektas A, et-al. Effect of activity and television viewing on BMI z-score in early adolescents in Turkey. World J Pediatr. 201;7:37–40.

264. Parvanta SA, Brown JD, Du S, et al. Television use and snacking behaviors among children and adolescents in China. J Adolesc Health 2010;46:339–45.

265. Adachi-Mejia AM, Longacre MR, Gibson JJ, et al. Children with a TV set in their bedroom at higher risk for being overweight. Int J Obes (Lond) 2007;31(4):644–51.

266. Barr-Anderson DJ, van den Berg P, Neumark-Sztainer D, et al. Characteristics associated with older adolescents. Pediatrics 2008;121:718–24.

267. Delmas C, Platat C, Schweitzer B, et al. Association between television in bedroom and adiposity throughout adolescence. Obesity (Silver Spring) 2007;15(10):2495–503.

268. Sisson SB, Broyles ST, Newton RL Jr, et al. TVs in the bedrooms of children: does it impact health and behavior? Prev Med 2011;52(2):104–8.

269. Stamatakis E, Hamer M, Dunstan DW. Screen-based entertainment time, all cause mortality, and cardiovascular events: population-based study with ongoing mortality and hospital events followup. J Am Coll Cardiol 2011;57(3):292–9.

270. Morrison JA, Glueck CJ, Daniels S, et al. Determinants of persistent obesity and hyperinsulinemia in a biracial cohort: a 15-year prospective study of schoolgirls. J Pediatr 2010;157:559–65.

271. Hardy LL, Denney-Wilson E, Thrift AP, et al. Screen time and metabolic risk factors among adolescents. Arch Pediatr Adolesc Med 2010;164:643–9.

272. Grøntved A, Hu FB. Television viewing and risk of type 2 diabetes, cardiovascular disease, and all-cause mortality: a meta-analysis. JAMA 2011;305(23):2448–55.

273. Mark AE, Janssen I. Relationship between screen time and metabolic syndrome in adolescents. J Public Health 2008;30(2):153–60.

274. Martinez-Gomez D, Tucker J, Heelan KA, et al. Associations between sedentary behavior and blood pressure in young children. Arch Pediatr Adolesc Med 2009;163:724–30.

275. Veerman JL, Healy GN, Cobiac LJ, et al. Television viewing time and reduced life expectancy: a life table analysis. Br J Sports Med 2011. Available at: http://press.psprings.co.uk/bjsm/august/bjsm85662.pdf. Accessed August 31, 2011.

276. Hardy LL, Bass SL, Booth ML. Changes in sedentary behavior among adolescent girls: a 2.5-year prospective cohort study. J Adolesc Health 2007;40:158–65.

277. Taveras EM, Field AE, Berkey CS, et al. Longitudinal relationship between television viewing and leisure-time physical activity during adolescence. Pediatrics 2007;119(2):e314–9.

278. Melkevik O, Torsheim T, Iannotti RJ, et al. Is spending time in screen-based sedentary behaviors associated with less physical activity: a cross national investigation. Int J Behav Nutr Phys Act 2010;7:46. Available at: http://www.ijbnpa.org/content/7/1/46. Accessed September 1, 2011.

279. Guthold R, Cowan MJ, Autenrieth CS, et al. Physical activity and sedentary behavior among schoolchildren: a 34-country comparison. J Pediatr 2010;157(1):43–9.

280. Cleland V, Venn A. Encouraging physical activity and discouraging sedentary behavior in children and adolescents. J Adolesc Health 2010;47:221–2.

281. Epstein LH, Roemmich JN, Cavanaugh MD, et al. The motivation to be sedentary predicts weight change when sedentary behaviors are reduced. Int J Behav Nutr Phys Act 2011;8:13. Available at: http://www.ijbnpa.org/content/pdf/1479-5868-8-13.pdf. Accessed August 31, 2011.

282. Leatherdale ST. Factors associated with communication-based sedentary behaviors among youth: are talking on the phone, texting, and instant messaging new sedentary behaviors to be concerned about? J Adolesc Health 2010;47:315–8.

283. Robinson TN. Reducing children's television viewing to prevent obesity: a randomized controlled trial. JAMA 1999;282(16):1561–7.

284. Epstein LH, Roemmich JN, Robinson JL, et al. A randomized trial of the effects of reducing television viewing and computer use on body mass index in young children. Arch Pediatr Adolesc Med 2008;162(3):239–45.

285. Maniccia DM, Davison KK, Marshall SJ, et al. A meta-analysis of interventions that target children's screen time for reduction. Pediatrics 2011;128(1):e193–210.

286. Graf DL, Pratt LV, Hester CN, et al. Playing active video games increases energy expenditure in children. Pediatrics 2009;124:534–40.

287. Daley AJ. Can exergaming contribute to improving physical activity levels and health outcomes in children? Pediatrics 2009;124:763–71.

288. Guy S, Ratzki-Leewing A, Gwadry-Sridhar G. Moving beyond the stigma: systematic review of video games and their potential to combat obesity. Int J Hypertens 2011. Available at: http://www.hindawi.com/journals/ijht/2011/179124/abs/. Accessed August 31, 2011.

289. Peng W, Lin JH, Crouse J. Is playing exergames really exercising? A meta-analysis of energy expenditure in active video games. Cyberpsychol Behav Soc Netw 2011. Available at: http://www.liebertonline.com/doi/abs/10.1089/cyber.2010.0578?journalCode=cyber. Accessed August 31, 2011.

290. Harris JL, Schwartz MB, Brownell KD, et al. Evaluating fast food nutrition and marketing to youth. New Haven (CT): Yale Rudd Center for Food Policy & Obesity; 2010.

291. Powell LM, Szczypka G, Chaloupka FJ, et al. Nutritional content of television food advertisements seen by children and adolescents in the United States. Pediatrics 2007;120(3):576–83.

292. Kunkel D, McKinley C, Stitt C. Food advertising during children's programming: a two-year comparison. Tucson (AZ): University of Arizona; 2010.

293. Gantz W, Schwartz N, Angelini JR, et al. Food for thought: television food advertising to children in the United States. Menlo Park (CA): Kaiser Family Foundation; 2007.

294. Sutherland LA, MacKenzie T, Purvis LA, et al. Prevalence of food and beverage brands in movies: 1996-2005. Pediatrics 2010;125:468–74.

295. Moore ES. It's child's play: advergaming and the online marketing of food to children. Menlo Park (CA): Kaiser Family Foundation; 2006.

296. Montgomery KC, Chester J. Interactive food and beverage marketing: targeting adolescents in the digital age. J Adolesc Health 2009;45(Suppl 3):S18–29.

297. Weber K, Story M, Harnack L. Internet food marketing strategies aimed at children and adolescents: a content analysis of food and beverage brand Web sites. J Am Diet Assoc 2006;106:1463–6.

298. Lee M, Choi Y, Quilliam ET, et al. Playing with food: content analysis of food advergames. J Consum Aff 2009;43:129–54.

299. Pempek TA, Calvert SL. Tipping the balance: use of advergames to promote consumption of nutritious foods and beverages by low-income African American children. Arch Pediatr Adolesc Med 2009;163:633–7.

300. Institute of Medicine. Preventing childhood obesity: health in the balance. Washington, DC: National Academies Press; 2005.

301. Robinson TN, Borzekowski DLG, Matheson DM, et al. Effects of fast food branding on young children's taste preferences. Arch Pediatr Adolesc Med 2007;161:792–7.

302. Federal Trade Commission. Interagency working group seeks input on proposed voluntary principles for marketing food to children. 2011. Available at: http://www.ftc.gov/opa/2011/04/foodmarket.shtm. Accessed September 1, 2011.

303. Layton L. Food makers resist lawmakers' proposal for guidelines in marketing to children. 2011. Available at: http://www.washingtonpost.com/politics/food-makers-resist-lawmakers-proposal-for-guidelines-in-marketing-to-children/2011/05/24/AFKf3mAH_story.html. Accessed September 1, 2011.

304. Kunkel D, McKinley C, Wright P. The impact of industry self-regulation on the nutritional quality of foods advertised on television to children. Oakland (CA): Children Now; 2009.

305. Koplan JP, Brownell KD. Response of the food and beverage industry to the obesity threat. JAMA 2010;13:1487–8.

306. Levi J, Segal LM, St. Laurent R, et al. F as in fat 2011: how obesity threatens America's future. Washington, DC: Robert Wood Johnson Foundation; 2011.

307. Blass EM, Anderson DR, Kirkorian HL, et al. On the road to obesity: television viewing increases intake of high-density foods. Physiol Behav 2006;88(4–5):597–604.

308. Utter J, Neumark-Sztainer D, Jeffery R, et al. Couch potatoes or French fries: Are sedentary behaviors associated with body mass index, physical activity, and dietary behaviors among adolescents? J Am Diet Assoc 2003;103:1298–305.

309. Vereecken CA, Todd J, Roberts C, et al. Television viewing behavior and associations with food habits in different countries. Public Health Nutr 2005;9:244–50.

310. Barr-Anderson DJ, Larson NI, Nelson MC, et al. Does television viewing predict dietary intake five years later in high school students and young adults? Int J

Behav Nutr Phys Act 2009;6:7. Available at: www.ijbnpa.org/content/6/1/7. Accessed August 31, 2011.

311. Strobele N, de Castro JM. Television viewing is associated with an increase in meal frequency in humans. Appetite 2004;42:111–3.

312. Wiecha JL, Peterson KE, Ludwig DS, et al. When children eat what they watch: impact of television viewing on dietary intake in youth. Arch Pediatr Adolesc Med 2006;160(4):436–42.

313. Harris JL, Bargh JA, Brownell KD. Priming effects of television food advertising on eating behavior. Health Psychol 2009;28(4):404–13.

314. Chamberlain LJ, Wang Y, Robinson TN. Does children's screen time predict requests for advertised products? Arch Pediatr Adolesc Med 2006;160:363–8.

315. Bell JF, Zimmerman FJ. Shortened nighttime sleep duration in early life and subsequent childhood obesity. Arch Pediatr Adolesc Med 2010;164(9):840–5.

316. Lytle LA, Pasch K, Farbaksh K. Is sleep related to obesity in young adolescents [abstract]? Presented at Pediatric Academic Societies meeting. Vancouver, British Columbia, Canada, May 2, 2010.

317. Garaulet M, Ortega FB, Ruiz JR, et al. Short sleep duration is associated with increased obesity markers in European adolescents: effect of physical activity and dietary habits. The HELENA study. Int J Obesity (Lond) 2011. Available at: http://www.nature.com/ijo/journal/vaop/ncurrent/full/ijo2011149a.html. Accessed September 1, 2011.

318. Taheri S. The link between short sleep duration and obesity: we should recommend more sleep to prevent obesity. Arch Dis Child 2006;91(11):881–4.

319. Johnson JG, Cohen P, Kasen S, et al. Association between television and sleep problems during adolescence and early adulthood. Arch Pediatr Adolesc Med 2004;158(6):562–8.

320. Dworak M, Schierl T, Bruns T, et al. Impact of singular excessive computer game and television exposure on sleep patterns and memory performance of school-aged children. Pediatrics 2007;120:978–85.

321. Wells TT, Cruess DG. Effects of partial sleep deprivation on food consumption and food choice. Psychol Health 2006;21(1):79–86.

322. Nelson MC, Gordon-Larsen P. Physical activity and sedentary behavior patterns are associated with selected adolescent health risk behaviors. Pediatrics 2006; 117(4):1281–90.

323. Van Cauter E, Holmback U, Knutson K, et al. Impact of sleep and sleep loss on neuroendocrine and metabolic function. Horm Res 2007;67(Suppl 1):2–9.

324. Higuchi S, Motohashi Y, Liu Y, et al. Effects of playing a computer game using a bright display on presleep physiological variables, sleep latency, slow wave sleep and REM sleep. J Sleep Res 2005;14(3):267–73.

325. Associated Press. More kids hospitalized for eating disorders. USA Today 2010. Available at: http://www.usatoday.com/yourlife/health/medical/pediatrics/2010-11-30-eating-disorders_N.htm. Accessed September 2, 2011.

326. Hogan MJ, Strasburger VC. Body image, eating disorders, and the media. Adolesc Med State Art Rev 2008;19(3):521–46.

327. Field AE, Javaras KM, Aneja P, et al. Family, peer, and media predictors of becoming eating disordered. Arch Pediatr Adolesc Med 2008;162(6):574–9.

328. Hayes S, Tantleff-Dunn S. Am I too fat to be a princess? Examining the effects of popular children's media on young girls' body image. Br J Dev Psychol 2010;28: 413–26.

329. Anschutz DJ, Spruijt-Metz D, Van Strien T, et al. The direct effect of thin ideal focused adult television on young girls' body figure. Body Image 2011;8:26–33.

330. Field AE, Camargo CA, Taylor CB, et al. Relation of peer and media influences to the development of purging behaviors among preadolescent and adolescent girls. Arch Pediatr Adolesc Med 1999;153(11):1184–9.

331. Abraham T. American Medical Association slams advertising industry for "exposing teens to bodies only attainable with the help of photo editing software." Daily Mail 2011. Available at: http://www.dailymail.co.uk/femail/article-2007532/American-Medical-Association-slams-advertising-industry-exposing-teens-bodies-attainable-help-photo-editing-software.html. Accessed September 2, 2011.

332. Martínez-Gonzalez MA, Gual P, Lahortiga F, et al. Parental factors, mass media influences, and the onset of eating disorders in a prospective population based cohort. Pediatrics 2003;111(2):315–20.

333. Moriarty CM, Harrison K. Television exposure and disordered eating among children: a longitudinal panel study. J Commun 2008;58:361–81.

334. Becker AE. Eating behaviours and attitudes following prolonged exposure to television among ethnic Fijian adolescent girls. Br J Psychiatry 2002;180:509–14.

335. Borzekowski DL, Schenk S, Wilson J, et al. e-Ana & e-Mia: a content analysis of pro-eating disorder Websites. Am J Public Health 2010;100:1526–34.

336. Becker AE, Fay KE, Agnew-Blaise J, et al. Social network media exposure and adolescent eating pathology in Fiji. Br J Psychiatry 2011;198:43–50.

337. Levine MP, Murnen SK. "Everybody knows that mass media are/are not [pick one] a cause of eating disorders": a critical review of evidence for a causal link between media, negative body image, and disordered eating in females. J Soc Clin Psychol 2009;28:9–42.

338. Nelson K. Structure and strategy in learning to talk. Monogr Soc Res Child Dev 1973;38(1-2):1–135. Serial 149.

339. Fisch SM, Truglio RT. "G" is for growing: thirty years of research on children and Sesame Street. Mahwah (NJ): Erlbaum; 2001.

340. Linebarger DL, Walker D. Infants' and toddlers' television viewing and language outcomes. Am Behav Sci 2005;48(5):624–5.

341. Tanimura M, Okuma K, Kyoshima K. Television viewing, reduced parental utterance, and delayed speech development in infants and young children. Arch Pediatr Adolesc Med 2007;161(6):618–9.

342. Zimmerman FJ, Christakis DA, Meltzoff AN. Associations between media viewing and language development in children under age 2 years. J Pediatr 2007;151(4):364–8.

343. Chonchaiya W, Pruksananonda C. Television viewing associates with delayed language development. Acta Paediatr 2008;97(7):977–82.

344. Mendelsohn AL, Berkule SB, Tomopoulos, et al. Infant television and video exposure associated with limited parent-child verbal interactions in low socioeconomic status households. Arch Pediatr Adolesc Med 2008;162:411–7.

345. Christakis DA, Gilkerson J, Richards J, et al. Audible television and decreased adult words, infant vocalizations, and conversational turns. Arch Pediatr Adolesc Med 2009;163(6):554–8.

346. Kirkorian HL, Pempek T, Murphy LA, et al. The impact of background television on parent-child interaction. Child Dev 2009;80:1350–9.

347. Schmidt ME, Rich M, Rifas-Shiman SL, et al. Television viewing in infancy and child cognition at 3 years of age in a US cohort. Pediatrics 2009;123:e370–5.

348. Richert RA, Robb MB, Fender JG, et al. Word learning from baby videos. Arch Pediatr Adolesc Med 2010;164:432–7.

349. Tomopoulos S, Dreyer BP, Berkule S, et al. Infant media exposure and toddler development. Arch Pediatr Adolesc Med 2010;164:1105–11.
350. DeLoache JS, Chiong C, Sherman K, et al. Do babies learn from baby media? Psychol Sci 2010;21:1570–4.
351. Krcmar M. Word learning in very young children from infant-directed DVDs. Journal of Communication 2011;61(4):780–94.
352. Brown A, Council on Communications and Media. Infant media use. Pediatrics 2011;128:1040–5.
353. Mendelsohn AL, Brockmeyer CA, Dreyer BP, et al. Do verbal interactions with infants during electronic media exposure mitigate adverse impacts on their language development as toddlers? Infant Child Dev 2010;19:577–93.
354. Richert R, Fender J. Parents' use of a DVD to teach toddlers' language. Presented at International Communication Association conference. Boston, MA, May 28, 2011.
355. Kuhl PK, Tsao FM, Liu HM. Foreign-language experience in infancy: effects of short-term exposure and social interaction on phonetic learning. Proc Natl Acad Sci U S A 2003;100:9096–101.
356. Christakis DA, Zimmerman FJ, DiGiuseppe DL, et al. Early television exposure and subsequent attentional problems in children. Pediatrics 2004;113(4):708–13.
357. Zimmerman FJ, Christakis DA. Associations between content types of early media exposure and attentional problems. Pediatrics 2007;120:986–92.
358. Swing EL, Gentile DA, Anderson CA, et al. Television and video game exposure and the development of attention problems. Pediatrics 2010;126:214–21.
359. Acevedo-Polakovich ID, Lorch EP, Milich R, et al. Disentangling the relation between television viewing and cognitive processes in children with attention deficit/hyperactivity disorder and comparison children. Arch Pediatr Adolesc Med 2006;160(4):354–60.
360. Chonchaiya W, Nuntnarumit P, Pruksananonda C. Comparison of television viewing between children with autism spectrum disorder and controls. Acta Paediatr 2011;100:1033–7.
361. Hancox RJ, Milne BJ, Poultn R. Association of television viewing during childhood with poor educational achievement. Arch Pediatr Adolesc Med 2005; 159(7):614–8.
362. Zimmerman FJ, Christakis DA. Children's television viewing and cognitive outcomes: a longitudinal analysis of national data. Arch Pediatr Adolesc Med 2005;159(7):619–25.
363. Borzekowski DL, Robinson TN. The remote, the mouse, and the No. 2 pencil: the household media environment and academic achievement among third grade students. Arch Pediatr Adolesc Med 2005;159(7):607–13.
364. Sharif I, Sargent JD. Association between television, movie, and video game exposure and school performance. Pediatrics 2006;118:e1061–70.
365. Sharif I, Wills TA, Sargent JA. Effect of visual media use on school performance: a prospective study. J Adolesc Health 2010;46:52–61.
366. Weis R, Cerankosky BC. Effects of video-game ownership on young boys' academic and behavioral functioning: a randomized, controlled study. Psychol Sci 2010. Available at: http://pss.sagepub.com/content/early/2010/02/17/0956797610362670.abstract. Accessed September 3, 2011.
367. Mossle T, Leimann M, Rehbein F, et al. Media use and school achievement—boys at risk? Br J Dev Psychol 2010;38(Pt 3):699–725.
368. Gould M, Jamieson P, Romer D. Media contagion and suicide among the young. Am Behav Sci 2003;46:1269–84.

369. Romer D, Jamieson PE, Jamieson KH. Are news reports of suicide contagious? A stringent test in six US cities. J Commun 2006;56(2):253–70.
370. Centers for Disease Control and Prevention (CDC): Guidelines for reporting suicide in the media. Available at: http://www.afsp.org/files/Misc_/recommendations.pdf. Accessed September 3, 2011.
371. Biddle L, Donovan J, Hawton K, et al. Suicide and the Internet. BMJ 2008;336: 800–2.
372. Dunlop SM, More E, Romer D. Where do youth learn about suicides on the Internet, and what influence does this have on suicidal ideation? J Child Psychol Psychiatry 2011. Available at: http://onlinelibrary.wiley.com/doi/10.1111/j.1469-7610.2011.02416.x/full. Accessed September 3, 2011.
373. Primack BA, Swanier B, Georgiopoulos AM, et al. Association between media use in adolescence and depression in young adulthood: a longitudinal study. Arch Gen Psychiatry 2009;66:181–8.
374. Kappos AD. The impact of electronic media on mental and somatic children's health. Int J Hyg Environ Health 2007;210:555–62.
375. Hamer M, Stamatakis E, Mishra G. Psychological distress, television viewing, and physical activity in children aged 4 to 12 years. Pediatrics 2009;123:1263–8.
376. Pagani LS, Fitzpatrick C, Barnett TA, et al. Prospective associations between early childhood television exposure and academic, psychosocial and physical well-being by middle childhood. Arch Pediatr Adolesc Med 2010;164:425–31.
377. Page AS, Cooper AR, Griew P, et al. Children's screen viewing is related to psychological difficulties irrespective of physical activity. Pediatrics 2010;126: e1011–7.
378. Lam LT, Peng Z- W. Effect of pathological use of the Internet on adolescent mental health. Arch Pediatr Adolesc Med 2010;164:901–6.
379. Hearold S. A synthesis of 1,043 effects of television on social behavior. In: Comstock G, editor. Public communication and behavior, vol. 1. New York: Academic Press; 1986. p. 65–133.
380. Mares L, Woodard E. Positive effects of television on children's social interactions: a meta-analysis. Media Psychol 2005;7(3):301–22.
381. Madsen K, Yen S, Wlasiuk L, et al. Feasibility of a dance videogame to promote weight loss among overweight children and adolescents. Arch Pediatr Adolesc Med 2007;161(1):105–7.
382. Bailey BW, McInnis K. Energy cost of exergaming. Arch Pediatr Adolesc Med 2011;165(7):597–602.
383. Sallis J. Potential vs. actual benefits of exergames. Arch Pediatr Adolesc Med 2011;165(7):667–9.
384. Graves LEF, Ridgers ND, Williams K, et al. The physiological cost and enjoyment of Wii Fit in adolescents, young adults, and older adults. J Phys Activ Health 2010;7(3):393–401.
385. Anderson D, Huston A, Schmitt K, et al. Early childhood television viewing and adolescent behavior: the Recontact Study. Monogr Soc Res Child Dev 2001; 66(1):1–147.
386. Crawley AM, Anderson DR, Santomero A, et al. Do children learn how to watch television? The impact of extensive experience with "Blue's Clues" on preschool children's television viewing behavior. J Commun 2002;5292:264–80.
387. Boyd D. Taken out of context: American teen sociality in networked publics [doctoral dissertation]. Berkeley (CA): University of California; 2008.
388. Kirkorian HL, Wartella EA, Anderson DR. Media and young children's learning. Future Child 2008;18(1):39–61.

389. Strasburger VC, Hogan MJ, Council on Communications and Media. Media education (policy statement). Pediatrics 2010;126(5):1012–7.
390. Rideout V. Parents, children, and media. Menlo Park (CA): Kaiser Family Foundation; 2007.
391. Jordan A, Hersey J, McDivitt J, et al. Reducing children's television-viewing time: a qualitative study of parents and their children. Pediatrics 2006;118(5): e1305–10, xxx.
392. Wahi G, Parkin PC, Beyene J, et al. Effectiveness of interventions aimed at reducing screen time in children. Arch Pediatr Adolesc Med 2011;165(11): 979–86.
393. Strasburger VC. Media and children: what need to happen now? JAMA 2009; 301(21):2265–6.
394. Longacre MR, Adachi-Mejia AM, Titus-Ernstoff L, et al. Parental attitudes about cigarette smoking and alcohol use in the Motion Picture Association of America rating system. Arch Pediatr Adolesc Med 2009;163(3):218–24.
395. Woodard E, Gridina N. Media in the home. Philadelphia: University of Pennsylvania Annenberg Public Policy Center; 2000.
396. O'Keefe GS, Clarke-Pearson K, Council on Communications and Media. Clinical report: the impact of social media on children, adolescents, and families. Pediatrics 2011;127:800–4.
397. Barkin SL, Finch SA, Ip EH, et al. Is office-based counseling about media use, timeouts, and firearm storage effective? Results from a cluster-randomized, controlled trial. Pediatrics 2008;122(1):e15–25.
398. Jackson C, Brown JD, Pardun CJ. A TV in the bedroom: implications for viewing habits and risk behaviors during early adolescence. J Broadcast Electronic Media 2008;52(3):349–67.
399. Strasburger VC. Children, adolescents, and the media: what we know, what we don't know, and what we need to find out (quickly!). Arch Dis Child 2009;94(9): 655–7.
400. Kirby D, Laris BA. Effective curriculum based sex and STD/HIV education programs for adolescents. Child Dev Perspect 2009;3(1):21–9.
401. McCannon B. Media literacy/media education: solution to big media? A review of the literature. In: Strasburger VC, Wilson BJ, Jordan A, editors. Children, adolescents, the media. 2nd edition. Thousand Oaks (CA): Sage; 2009. p. 519–69.
402. Rosenkoetter LI, Rosenkoetter SE, Acock AC. Television violence: an intervention to reduce its impact on children. J Appl Dev Psychol 2008;30(4):381–97.
403. Primack BA, Hobbs R. Association of various components of media literacy and adolescent smoking. Am J Health Behav 2009;33(2):192–201.
404. Primack BA, Sidani J, Carroll MV, et al. Associations between smoking and media literacy in college students. J Health Commun 2009;14(6):541–55.
405. Strasburger VC. School daze: why are teachers and schools missing the boat on media? Pediatr Clin North Am 2012. [Epub ahead of print].
406. Up in smoke: Disney bans cigarettes. ABCnews.com; 2007. Available at: http://abcnews.go.com/GMA/story?id=3416434&page=1. Accessed December 1, 2011.
407. American Academy of Pediatrics, Committee on Communications. Children, adolescents, and advertising. Pediatrics 2006;118(6):2563–9.
408. Brownell KD, Schwartz MB, Puhl RM, et al. The need for bold action to prevent adolescent obesity. J Adolesc Health 2009;45(3S):S8–17.
409. Stitt C, Kunkel D. Food advertising during children's television programming on broadcast and cable channels. Health Commun 2008;23(6):573–84.

410. Jordan A, Kramer-Golinkoff E, Strasburger VC. Do the media cause obesity and eating disorders? Adolesc Med State Art Rev 2008;19(3):431–49.
411. Jordan AB, Robinson TN. Children, television viewing, and weight status: summary and recommendations from an expert panel meeting. Ann Am Acad Pol Soc Sci 2008;615(1):119–32.
412. Harris JL, Pomeranz JL, Lobstein T, et al. A crisis in the marketplace: how food marketing contributes to childhood obesity and what can be done. Annu Rev Public Health 2009;30:211–25.
413. Ofcom. Children watching fewer TV adverts for less healthy foods, review finds. 2008. Available at: http://media.ofcom.org.uk/2008/12/17/children-watching-fewer-tv-adverts-for-less-healthy-foods-review-finds/. Accessed December 1, 2011.
414. Dixon HG, Scully ML, Wakefield MA, et al. The effects of television advertisements for junk food versus nutritious food on children's food attitudes and preferences. Soc Sci Med 2007;65(7):1311–23.
415. Livingstone S, Haddon L, Gorzig A, et al. EU Kids Online: Final report. LSE. London: EU Kids Online; 2011. Available at: http://www2.lse.ac.uk/media@lse/research/EUKidsOnline/Home.aspx. Accessed December 1, 2011.
416. Simon M. Junk food industry determined to target kids. 2011. Available at: http://www.foodsafetynews.com/2011/07/junk-food-industry-determined-to-target-kids/. Accessed December 1, 2011.
417. Speers SE, Harris JL, Schwartz MB. Child and adolescent exposure to food and beverage brand appearances during prime-time television programming. Am J Prev Med 2011;41(3):291–6.
418. Wilson BJ, Kunkel D, Drogos KL. Educationally/insufficient? An analysis of the availability & educational quality of children's E/I programming. Oakland (CA): Children Now; 2008. Available at: http://www.childrennow.org/uploads/documents/eireport_2008.pdf. Accessed December 1, 2011.
419. Eggerton J. FCC to revisit kids TV rules. Broadcast Cable. 2009. Available at: http://www.broadcastingcable.com/article/316123-FCC_To_Revisit_Kids_TV_Rules.php Accessed December 1, 2011.
420. Christakis DA, Zimmerman FJ. Media as a public health issue. Arch Pediatr Adolesc Med 2006;160:445–6.

Overview: New Media

Gwenn Schurgin O'Keeffe, MD

KEYWORDS

- New media • Web 1.0 • Web 2.0 • Digital divide • Participatory culture
- Social media • Digital families • Pediatricians

KEY POINTS

- Technology is influential in children's lives from a very young age, especially new media, which occur on everything children use today.
- Technology can cause health problems when issues such as sexting, cyberbullying, and privacy breaches develop.
- Pediatricians must be well versed in new media to adequately care for today's children.
- All generations use new media, although slightly differently.
- Knowing what new media each age group uses helps pediatricians ask the right questions to detect issues like cyberbullying and sexting.

For the very first time the young are seeing history being made before it is censored by their elders.

—Margaret Mead[1]

Social media is like teen sex. Everyone wants to do it. No one actually knows how. When finally done, there is surprise it's not better.
—Avinash Kaushik, Google's analytics evangelist via Twitter[2]

Pediatricians have a difficult task: to care for children's growth and development from the time they are born until they become adults. In addition to physical, emotional, and developmental growth, pediatricians also must be vigilant for external influences, which can have a profound impact on health and well being.[3] In today's society, one of the most influential factor's on children of all ages is technology, as shown by the common sights of children using cell phones, listening to MP3 players, and using laptops and handheld devices. Seventy-five percent of teenagers own cell phones, with 25% using them for social media.[4] According to Common Sense Media, 22% of teenagers log onto their favorite social media site more than 10 times a day.[5]

Pediatrics Now, PO Box 5336, Wayland, MA 01778, USA
E-mail address: drgwenn@pediatricsnow.com

Pediatr Clin N Am 59 (2012) 589–600
doi:10.1016/j.pcl.2012.03.024
0031-3955/12/$ – see front matter © 2012 Elsevier Inc. All rights reserved.

With the increase in technology comes not only an increase in skills and social bene-fits, but the potential for harm such as sexting, cyberbullying, privacy issues, and Internet addiction, all of which may present with vague health symptoms.[6] Therefore, it is crucial for pediatricians to become well versed in the new media their patients and families are using. That is the only way to provide media-oriented anticipatory guid-ance and advice on media-related issues when they arise.

NEW MEDIA DEFINED

Media today include many different forms. At their core, they are all forms of commu-nication. Media that evolved before digital technology have come to be known as traditional media, whereas media that have evolved since the development of digital technology are known as new media.

Examples of traditional media include all print materials, radio, television, records, and cassettes. Media consumption in this category tend to be passive. People are given these media; they do not create them or interact with them.[7]

New media include everything that is now used on a device or computer. E-readers, smartphones, computers, laptops, CDs, DVDs, MP3 players, and everything they produce are new media. Media consumption in this category is social and active. People can respond to these media and interact with them, if they choose to.[8]

New media technologies are further subclassified by their evolution in the digital world. Web 1.0 typically refers to Internet sites using the earliest web-based technol-ogies, whereas 2.0 sites refer to sites that are the newest and are using the most social tools. The differences between the 1.0 media and 2.0 or new media have to do with the purpose of the sites and the user experiences. Web 1.0 sites are passive, whereas 2.0 sites are active (**Table 1**).

Table 1
Comparison of Web 1.0 and Web 2.0 Web sites. Created by Gwenn O'Keeffe, MD, FAAP based on material from http://www.darrenbarefoot.com/archives/2006/05/web-10-vs-web-20.htm

Web 1.0	Web 2.0
1. Static	1. Dynamic
2. Home pages	2. Blogs
3. Reading	3. Writing
4. Companies	4. Communities
5. HTML	5. XML
6. Client server	6. Peer to peer
7. Lectures	7. Conversation
8. Advertising	8. Word of mouth
9. Wires	9. Wireless
10. Dial-up access	10. Broadband access
11. All about ownership	11. All about sharing
12. Netscape for search	12. Google for search
13. Owning	13. Sharing
14. Internet Explorer browser	14. Firefox browser
15. Like a newspaper	15. Like TV/video
16. Considered a tool	16. Considered a lifestyle

IMPACT ON SOCIETY

The major impact of new media extends beyond technological advances and into the fiber of our society. New media, particularly the more recent advances online, have pushed our society toward a more participatory culture.[9] According to Henry Jenkins, "[a] participatory culture is culture with relatively low barriers to artistic expression and civic engagement, strong support for creating and sharing one's creations, and some type of informal mentorship whereby what is known by the most experienced is passed along to novices. A participatory culture is also one in which members believe their contributions matter, and feel some degree of social connection with one another...."[9]

New media allow people to thrive in a participatory culture and enjoy benefits such as peer-to-peer collaboration, cultural diversity, enhanced learning, and more engaged citizens. In addition, with new media, people are more connected to their health and health care systems.[6,9]

Use of new media and how each generation uses new media shows how participatory our society has become. According to the most recent data from Pew Internet and American Life Project (**Fig. 1**), adults and teens are both online, but teens are online more than adults. However, both share similarities in the activities they do online, such as reading news, engaging in e-mail, shopping, and watching videos. Although

Survey dates for online activities charts

Activity	Online teens	Teen Survey Date	Online adults	Adult Survey Date
Go online	93%	Sep-09	79%	May-10
% of internet users who do the following activities:				
Send or read e-mail	73	Sep-09	94	May-10
Use a search engine	*	*	87	May-10
Get news	62~	Sep-09	75	May-10
Visit a government website	*	*	67	May-10
Buy a product	48	Sep-09	66	May-10
Make travel reservations	*	*	66	May-10
Watch a video	57	Nov-06	66	May-10
Use social networking sites	73	Sep-09	61	May-10
Bank online	*	*	58	May-10
Use online classifieds	*	*	53	May-10
Send instant messages	67	Sep-09	47	May-10
Get financial info	*	*	38	May-10
Look for religious/spiritual info	*	*	32	May-10
Rate a product, service or person	*	*	32	May-10
Participate in an auction	*	*	26	May-10
Make a charitable donation	*	*	22	May-10
Download podcasts	*	*	21	May-10
Work on own blog	14	Sep-09	14	Jan-10
Listen to music online	*	*	51	Sept-09
Visit a virtual world	8	Sep-09	4	Sept-09
Look for health info	31~	Sep-09	83	Dec-08
Read blogs	49	Nov-06	32	Dec-08
Play online games	78	Feb-08	35^	Aug-06

Note: ~ indicates significant differences in question wording between teen data and adult data.

Fig. 1. Breakdown in online activities between teen and adult users. In general, the online activities are similar between the 2 groups. (*Courtesy of* Pew Internet & American Life Project; with permission.)

adults search for health information more than teens, one-third of teens go online for health information.[10]

However, the generational differences become more pronounced among the adult groups, as shown in **Fig. 2**, with the oldest populations least involved in all online activities compared with the younger generations of adults, and with teens.

Within the teen generation, a 2009 Pew Internet survey showed that not all teenagers use the Internet to the same degree as noted in **Fig. 3**. However, despite slight socioeconomic and racial differences in how teens use digital devices, data show that most teens are online (**Fig. 3**).

NEW MEDIA AND TODAY'S FAMILY
The Digital American Family

Context is everything in evaluating a child. Illnesses that a child may come in contact with, stress, and peers all matter in influencing the health of a child. A child's digital life plays a role as well.

Knowing how digital today's family has become helps the health care services help them with media-related issues. It also helps health care services know where to begin in learning about new media, technologically, and in anticipating the issues that may arise from the use of that technology by children, teens, and parents.

Activity	Teens Ages 12-17	Millennials Ages 18-33	Gen X Ages 34-45	Younger Boomers Ages 46-55	Older Boomers Ages 56-64	Silent Gen Ages 65-73	G.I. Gen Age 74+	All adults Age 18+
Go online	93%	95%	86%	81%	76%	58%	30%	79%
Teens and/or Millennials are more likely to engage in the following activities compared with older users:								
Watch a video	57	80	66	62	55	44	20	66
Use social network sites	73	83	62	50	43	34	16	61
Send instant messages	67	66	52	35	30	29	4	47
Play online games	78	50^	38^	26^	28^	25^	18^	35^
Read blogs	49^	43	34	27	25	23	15	32
Visit a virtual world	8	4	4	4	3	3	1	4

Note: ^ indicates data from 2006.
Source: Pew Research Center's Internet & American Life Project surveys , 2008-2010. All teens data are from different surveys than adult data, and may have slight differences in question wording. Findings for individual activities are based on internet users. For survey dates of all activities cited, please see the Methodology section at the end of this report.

Fig. 2. Generational breakdown of adult online use with a difference between younger and older adult use patterns. (*Courtesy of* Pew Internet & American Life Project; with permission.)

Demographics of teen internet users

Below is the percentage of teens in each group who use the internet, according to our September 2009 survey. As an example, 94% of teen girls use the internet.

	% who use the internet
Total teens	93
Boys	91
Girls	94
Race/ethnicity	
White, Non-Hispanic	94
Black, Non-Hispanic	87
Hispanic (English -speaking)	95
Age	
12-13	88
14-17	95
Household income	
Less than $30,000/yr	88
$30,000-$49,999	89
$50,000-$74,999	96
$75,000+	97

Source: The Pew Research Center's Internet & American Life project 2009 Parent-Teen Cell Phone Survey, conducted from June 26 to September 24, 2009. n= 800 teens ages 12-17 (including 245 cell phone interviews).

pewinternet.org

Fig. 3. Demographic and racial differences in teen online use. (*Courtesy of* Pew Internet & American Life Project; with permission.)

According to Nielsen's *The New Digital American Family*, "(t)he New Digital American Family is getting older, smaller, growing more slowly and becoming more ethnically diverse than at any point in history. Diversity in all its dimensions defines the emerging American Family archetype, with no single cultural, social, demographic, economic or political point of view dominating the landscape."[11]

According to Nielsen, most of today's parents are from Generation X. Born between 1965 and 1976, this group represents 43.9% of homes with children less than 18 years of age. The next largest group is the Brady Boomers. Born between 1956 and 1964, this group comprises 23.3% of parents. Baby Boomers, born between 1946 and 1964, still represent a sizable force in the parenting generation, representing nearly 30%.[11]

Matching this information with the Pew Generations chart mentioned earlier, health care services can fine tune the way families are questioned.

Teens and Adults

Pew and others have shown that search, social media, e-mail, and video are the main destinations online for all generations, but to what extent? What sites attention be focused on?

Data by Experian Hitwise from the week of December 3, 2011 help answer these questions, as noted in **Fig. 4**. The top 4 items on this chart represent the top 4 activities that are known to be important to all generations:

- Facebook: social media
- Google: search

Top 10 visited US websites

The following report shows **websites** for the industry **'All Categories'**, ranked by **Visits** for the **week** ending **12/03/2011**.

Rank	Website	Visits Share	
1.	Facebook	9.03%	
2.	Google	7.15%	
3.	YouTube	2.89%	
4.	Yahoo! Mail	2.69%	
5.	Yahoo!	2.45%	
6.	Bing	1.39%	
7.	Yahoo! Search	1.34%	
8.	Gmail	1.23%	
9.	msn	0.98%	
10.	Windows Live Mail	0.89%	

Fig. 4. Most visited US Web sites in December 2011. (*Courtesy of* Experian Hitwise; with permission.)

- YouTube: video
- Yahoo! Mail: e-mail

Teasing through the social media sites further, other sites emerge as popular players in this field (**Fig. 5**):

What is interesting about **Fig. 5** is that Google+ is already in the top 10 and is new to the social media landscape. Being able to track this sort of trend will be helpful in knowing where families may be getting information online and, hence, what to ask them about.

The total number of users on these sites is staggering. As of June 2011, Facebook had 734 million users a month and Twitter 144 million users a month.[12] Among teens,

Top 10 Social Networking sites

The following report shows **websites** for the industry **'Computers and Internet - Social Networking and Forums'**, ranked by **Visits** for the **week** ending **12/03/2011**.

Rank	Website	Visits Share	
1.	Facebook	63.63%	
2.	YouTube	20.36%	
3.	Twitter	1.52%	
4.	Yahoo! Answers	1.02%	
5.	Tagged	0.74%	
6.	Linkedin	0.65%	
7.	Google+	0.58%	
8.	MySpace	0.47%	
9.	myYearbook	0.41%	
10.	Pinterest.com	0.34%	

Fig. 5. Top 10 social networking sites, December 2011. (*Courtesy of* Experian Hitwise; with permission.)

73% use social media sites such as these.[13] Although Facebook is popular among teens, as it is with adults, Twitter is not, with only 8% of teens actively using Twitter.[13]

In a clinical encounter, knowing what sites families are spending time on is how they can be helped to make more healthy choices as well as to navigate issues when they occur. For example, by being aware that people spend most of their online time on Facebook and YouTube (**Fig. 5**), time can be focused on helping families understand those sites.

Similar trends reported by NM Incite show that parents use social media for similar reasons as teens: entertainment, gaming, connection.[14] Cell phone use and the accessing of new media via cell phones are increasing; 75% of teens and 93% of adults own cell phones.[13] All of these activities are important in monitoring and counseling families in the clinical setting.

Today's family is digitally savvy, an observation confirmed not just by Pew and Experian but other groups such as Nielsen.[11] "For members of the Post-Digital Generation, there has always been an Internet. Time-shifted viewing has become the norm. Three-screen lifestyles (TV, Internet and mobile) predominate. Social media use continues to soar... The Internet is more than a way to study."[11]

Children Aged 0 to 13 Years

Teens and adults are not the only populations using new media. Children as young as toddlers are now exposed to new media technologies. According to Common Sense Media,[15] the total screen time for this population is significant. According to their recent report, *Zero to Eight: Children's Media Use in America*, people in this age group spend 27% of their time with digital devices, which includes computers, video games, tablets, cell phones, and other handheld and mobile devices.

Other important data for this age group:

- 52% have access to some sort of mobile device, such as a cell phone or smart phone[15]
- All children in this age bracket use computers: 53% of children aged 2 to 4 years and 90% of children aged 5 to 8 years[15]
- In the 2- to 5-year-old age group[16]
  - 58% can play a basic computer game
  - 19% can use a Smartphone App but only 11% can tie their shoelaces
- More children aged 2 and 3 years can play a computer game than ride a bike (58% vs 52%).[17]

Studies confirm what is seen in society: media use increases with age. Compared with the toddlers and preschoolers, the later elementary school group, children aged 6 to 9 years, are online even more[17] with:

- One-fifth using e-mail
- 14% using Facebook despite the registration age being 13 years
- 47% talking with friends online
- US children logging 4 hours of Internet time weekly, 30 minutes more than the international average.

By 11 years of age, most US tweens are on new media sites such as Twitter or Facebook; 62% of the group aged 10 and 13 years are actively using social media.[18]

Most children aged 10 to 13 years, both in the United States and internationally, report having their own computers.[18]

NEW MEDIA AND PEDIATRICS

Pediatricians use new media in a similar way as their patients, as shown[19] in **Fig. 6**. These data are consistent with other generational data and help explain how technology is used both personally and professionally.[10] Similarly, pediatricians, like the general public, are heavy social media users (**Fig. 7**), and this tracks along generational lines.[10]

NEW MEDIA AND THE FUTURE

To keep up with new media trends, pediatricians are best served by using their own new media use as one guide and the new media their patients are using as another guide. Knowing that their use is similar to their patients' and families' use should help them find common ground to help discuss technology issues and intervene when necessary.

In addition, the American Academy of Pediatrics' *Talking to Children and Teens about Social Media and Sexting* is not only a helpful guide for parents but also for pediatricians. The advice for social media does not just apply to sites such as Facebook but to any new media venue or technology:

- Let them know that their use of technology is something you want and need to know about. For kids of all ages, ask daily: "Have you used the computer and the Internet today?
  - Technology use varies by age. Tweens are likely to be using more instant messaging (IM) and texting, whereas teens use those technologies and also networking sites such as Facebook. (These tools often are referred to as platforms for social networking.) Ask daily how your family used those tools with questions such as: What did you write on Facebook today? Any new chats recently? Anyone text you today?
  - Share a bit about your daily social media use as a way to facilitate daily conversation about your children's online habits.
  - Get your children talking about their social media lives so that you know what they are doing.

Ways pediatricians use the Internet by age group, 2009 (% using)				
	30s, n=205	40s, n=208	50s, n=224	60s, n=105
Get news**	95%	94%	85%	88%
Earn CME**	74	76	67	55
Watch videos (YouTube)**	74	76	67	58
Read blogs or journals*	44	33	30	34
Download podcasts	29	30	29	23
Create blog or journal	15	10	11	6
Use Twitter	13	9	8	4

*$P<.05$, **$P<.01$

Fig. 6. Ways pediatricians use the Internet by age group, showing similarities among generations of pediatricians. American Academy of Pediatrics, Periodic Survey of Fellows No. 75, 2009. (*From* the American Academy of Pediatrics, Periodic Survey of Fellows No. 75, 2009. Reprinted with permission of AAP News, June 2010.)

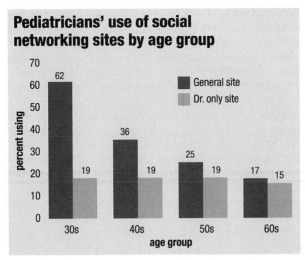

Pediatricians' use of social networking sites by age group

Fig. 7. Pediatrician social media use. American Academy of Pediatrics, Periodic Survey of Fellows No. 75, 2009. (*From* the American Academy of Pediatrics, Periodic Survey of Fellows No. 75, 2009. Reprinted with permission of AAP News, June 2010.)

- Keep the computer in a public part of your home, such as the family room or kitchen, so that you can check on what your children are doing online and how much time they are spending there.
- Talk with other parents about what their children of similar ages are using for social media. Ask your children about those technologies as a starting point for discussion. If they are in the same peer group, there is a good chance that they are all using the same platforms together. For example
  - For teens: Mrs Smith told me that Jennifer uses Facebook. Is that something you have thought of doing? Do you already have a profile? If so, I would like to see it.
  - For tweens and older elementary school children: Are you planning on meeting up with children on Club Penguin today? I would love to see how that works. Or, Let's look at your text log today together. I would like to see who has been texting you.

For all ages, emphasize that everything sent over the Internet or a cell phone can be shared with the world, so it is important that they use good judgment in sending messages and pictures and set privacy settings on social media sites appropriately.

- Discuss with children of every age what good judgment means and the consequences of poor judgment, ranging from minor punishment to possible legal action in the case of sexting (discussed later) or bullying.
- Remember to make a point of discouraging children from gossiping, spreading rumors, bullying or damaging someone's reputation using texting or other tools.
- To keep children safe, have your children and teens show you where the privacy features are for every social media venue they are using. The more private they are, the less likely it is that inappropriate material will be received by your child, or be sent to their circle of acquaintances.
- Be aware of the ages of use for sites that your tweens and older elementary school children want to use, including game sites such as Club Penguin and Webkinz. Many sites are for age 13 years and older, and the sites for younger children require parental consent to use.

- Be sure you are where your children are online: IM, Facebook, MySpace, and so forth. Have a policy requiring that you and your child friend each other. This is one way of showing your child that you are there, too, and will provide a checks-and-balance system by having an adult within arm's reach of their profile. This precaution is important for children of all ages, including teens.
- Show your children that you know how to use what they are using, and are willing to learn what you may not know how to do.
- Create a strategy for monitoring your children's online social media use, and be sure you follow through. Some families may check once a week and others more sporadically. You may want to say, "Today I'll be checking your computer and cell phone." The older your children are, the more often you may need to check.
- Consider formal monitoring systems to track your child's e-mail, chat, IM, and image content. Parental controls on your computer or from your Internet service provider, Google Desktop, or commercial programs are all reasonable alternatives.
- Set time limits for Internet and cell phone use. Learn the warning signs of trouble: skipping activities, meals, and homework for social media; weight loss or gain; a reduction in grades. If these issues are occurring because of your children being online when they should be eating, sleeping, or participating in school or social activities, your children may have a problem with Internet or social media addiction. Contact your pediatrician for advice if any of these symptoms are occurring.
- Check chat logs, e-mails, files, and social networking profiles for inappropriate content, friends, messages, and images periodically. Be transparent and let your children know what you are doing.
- Multitasking can be dangerous, even deadly. Be sure to stress to teens the importance of not texting, using Facebook, using the phone, listening to ear buds or earphones, or engaging in similarly distracting activities while driving. These forms of distracted driving are illegal in many states because they are so dangerous. In addition, caution children of all ages about using mobile devices while walking, biking, babysitting, or doing other things that require their full attention.[20]

Pediatricians are uniquely positioned to help families understand how the digital world affects a child's health and development. For that reason, the American Academy of Pediatrics has issued a clinical report on social media for pediatricians with the following advice[6]:

Pediatricians are in a unique position to educate families about both the complexities of the digital world and the challenging social and health issues that online youth experience by encouraging families to face the core issues of bullying, popularity and status, depression and social anxiety, risk-taking, and sexual development. Pediatricians can help parents understand that what is happening online is an extension of these underlying issues and that parents can be most helpful if they understand the core issues and have strategies for dealing with them whether they take place online, offline, or, increasingly, both.

Some specific ways in which pediatricians can assist parents include

1. Advise parents to talk to their children and adolescents about their online use and the specific issues that today's online kids face.

2. Advise parents to work on their own participation gap in their homes by becoming better educated about the many technologies their youngsters are using.

3. Discuss with families the need for a family online-use plan that involves regular family meetings to discuss online topics and checks of privacy settings and online profiles for inappropriate posts. The emphasis should be on citizenship and healthy behavior and not punitive action, unless warranted.

4. Discuss with parents the importance of supervising online activities via active participation and communication,as opposed to remote monitoring with a "net-nanny" program (software used to monitor the Internet in the absence of parents).

Pediatricians are already more technologically savvy than they realize. With better communication and recognition of how their families use new media, they can better incorporate new media technologies into all areas of pediatric practice from general care to subspecialty practices.

REFERENCES

1. Brainy Quote. Margaret Mead. Available at: http://www.brainyquote.com/quotes/authors/m/margaret_mead.html. Accessed December 7, 2011.
2. McCarthy C. Cnet News: Quote of the day is like teen sex. Available at: http://news.cnet.com/8301-13577_3-10185477-36.html. Accessed December 7, 2011.
3. Behrman RE, Kliegman RM, Nelson WE, et al. The field of pediatrics. Nelson textbook of pediatrics. Philadelphia: Saunders; 1992.
4. Lenhart A. Teens and sexting. Washington, DC: Pew Research Center; 2009. Available at: http://pewinternet.org/Reports/2009/Teens-and-Sexting.aspx. Accessed January 3, 2012.
5. Common Sense Media. Is technology networking changing childhood? A national poll. San Francisco (CA): Common Sense Media; 2009. Available at: www.commonsensemedia.org/sites/default/files/CSM_teen_social_media_080609_FINAL.pdf. Accessed January 3, 2012.
6. O'Keeffe GS. The impact of social media on children, adolescents, and families. Pediatrics 2011. Available at: http://pediatrics.aappublications.org/content/127/4/800.full?sid=8d594369-3d6b-4852-a2b7-8aab26c96a88. Accessed December 7, 2011.
7. Definition: traditional media. PCMag.com. Available at: http://www.pcmag.com/encyclopedia_term/0,t=old+media&i=56879,00.asp,2542. Accessed December 7, 2011.
8. Definition: new media. PCMag.com. Available at: http://www.pcmag.com/encyclopedia_term/0,2542,t=new+media&i=47936,00.asp. Accessed December 7, 2011.
9. Jenkins H. YouTube TedEx NY. Available at: http://www.youtube.com/watch?v=AFCLKaOXRlw&feature=player_embedded#!. Accessed December 9, 2011.
10. Zickuhr, Kathryn. Generations 2010. Pew Research Center's Internet & American Life Project. Pew Research Center's Internet & American Life Project; 2012. Available at: http://pewinternet.org/Reports/2010/Generations-2010.aspx. Accessed January 3, 2012.
11. Anderson D, Subramanyam R. Rep New Digital American Family. New York (NY): The Nielsen Company; 2011.
12. Marketing data, HubSpot marketing reports. Available at: http://blog.hubspot.com/blog/tabid/6307/bid/14715/12-Essential-Facebook-Stats-Data.aspx. Accessed December 19, 2011.

13. Lenhart A. Social media and young adults. Washington, DC: Pew Research Center; 2010. Available at: http://www.pewinternet.org/Reports/2010/Social-Media-and-Young-Adults.aspx. Accessed January 3, 2012.

14. Parenting use of social media. HubSpot marketing reports. Available at: http://blog.hubspot.com/blog/tabid/6307/bid/14715/12-Essential-Facebook-Stats-Data.aspx. Accessed December 19, 2011.

15. Rideout VJ. Zero to eight: children's media use in America. Common Sense Media report. 2011.

16. Stage two. Digital diaries. 2012. Available at: http://www.avgdigitaldiaries.com/tagged/stage_two. Accessed January 3, 2012.

17. Stage three. Digital diaries. 2012. Available at: http://www.avgdigitaldiaries.com/tagged/stage_three. Accessed January 3, 2012.

18. Stage four. Digital diaries. 2012. Available at: http://www.avgdigitaldiaries.com/tagged/stage_four. Accessed January 3, 2012.

19. Periodic survey explores age gap in pediatricians' use of Internet, social media. American Academy of Pediatrics News. June 1, 2010. Available at: http://aapnews.aappublications.org/content/31/6/13.1.full.pdf+html. Accessed December 7, 2011.

20. Talking to kids and teens about social media and sexting. American Academy of Pediatrics. Available at: http://www.aap.org/en-us/about-the-aap/aap-press-room/news-features-and-safety-tips/Pages/Talking-to-Kids-and-Teens-About-Social-Media-and-Sexting.aspx. Accessed December 19, 2011.

Social Networking Sites and Adolescent Health

Megan A. Moreno, MD, MSEd, MPH[a],*, Jennifer Kolb, MD[b]

KEYWORDS

- Adolescent • Social networking site • Facebook • Professionalism

KEY POINTS

- Social networking sites (SNSs) allow users to create a personal Web profile and communicate with and build an online social network.
- Risks to SNSs include display of risky material and privacy violations; SNSs can also be a venue for cyberbullying or sexting.
- Benefits of SNSs include access to support, improved self-esteem and social capital, and organization of classroom or civic activities.
- Pediatricians have unique risks and benefits when using SNSs given their roles as professionals.

LOL, OMG, TTYL, KIT, and *TTFN*: these terms may look and sound like a strange new foreign language, and in some ways, they are. Chances are, however, the average 10 year old could translate them within a matter of seconds. Adolescents today have grown up in a world of technology, with iPads, smartphones, and SNSs at their fingertips. Parents and other adults are slowly catching up in terms of technological knowledge; however, it seems there is a still a large gap between the ease with which adolescents are able to manipulate technology and the ease with which their parents can. In recent years there has been a significant increase in research investigating the potential risks and benefits of these new technologies. The knowledge gained from these studies can benefit every adolescent, parent, and even pediatrician.

The majority of adolescents today have Internet access, with some youth reporting up to 10 hours of media use per day.[1] A popular online activity for adolescents is creating and maintaining personal profiles on SNSs. SNSs are Web sites that allow users to share information about themselves and their lives with large groups of people. Members are able to create a profile with demographic information as well as interests and hobbies, upload pictures and videos, join groups about topics they

[a] Department of Pediatrics, University of Wisconsin–Madison, 2870 University Avenue, Suite 200, Madison, WI 53705, USA; [b] Department of Pediatrics, University of Wisconsin–Madison, 600 Highland Avenue, H4/444, Madison, WI 53792, USA
* Corresponding author.
E-mail address: mamoreno@pediatrics.wisc.edu

Pediatr Clin N Am 59 (2012) 601–612
doi:10.1016/j.pcl.2012.03.023   pediatric.theclinics.com
0031-3955/12/$ – see front matter © 2012 Elsevier Inc. All rights reserved.

are interested in, post comments (called *status updates*) about recent events, communicate with friends via e-mail or instant messages, and link their profiles with others in a process referred to as *friending*.[2,3] For adolescents, SNSs are an important medium for self-expression, communication with friends, and peer feedback.[3] One study reported that 73% of teens between ages 12 and 17 owned an SNS profile, whereas another study found that 22% of teenagers log onto their favorite SNSs more than 10 times per day.[4] Even younger children are participating in SNS activities; one study found that 20% of youth ages 8 to 10 used an SNS daily.[5]

There are different types of SNSs available on the Internet, some with a more targeted audience than others. The more common SNSs used by adolescents include Facebook, Myspace, and Twitter. Other SNSs are available for professional networking targeted at adult populations (eg, LinkedIn) or for interactive learning aimed at younger children (eg, Disney).

FACEBOOK

Facebook (www.facebook.com) originated in 2004 as a Harvard University Web site for students of that university to connect and communicate.[2] Since then, it has expanded over time to its current status such that anyone over age 13 can register for and create a profile page (Congress passed the Children's Online Privacy Protection Act, which prohibits Web sites from collecting information from individuals under age 13).[6] The mission of Facebook, as posted on its Web site is "to give people the power to share and make the world more open and connected."[6] As of July 2011, there were 800 million users worldwide, and, recently, Facebook has replaced Google as the Web site with the most daily visits.[7] It is also currently the most popular SNS among adolescents. A 2009 study found that of 1828 high school students who owned an SNS profile, 68.5% preferred Facebook to any other site.[8]

MYSPACE

Myspace (www.myspace.com) was launched in 2003 and quickly gained global popularity. Myspace grew as a site where users can personalize a profile page, post blog and journal entries, and communicate with friends, with a focus on discovering and sharing new music.[4] The popularity of Myspace, however, has continually declined since 2008. In 2006, the estimated number of profiles that were invalid or deleted was 6.4%, whereas the number in 2009 was 44.1%.[4] Also, the 2009 study of 1828 high school students who owned SNS profiles found that only 13% preferred Myspace to other SNSs.[8] As further evidence of its decline, in 2010, Myspace was the seventh most popular Web site in the United States, but as of December 2011, it ranked 135th in total Web traffic.[4,9] The rise and decline of Myspace illustrates that not all popular SNSs have longevity. Many Myspace profile owners switched to Facebook, however, because this site skyrocketed in popularity. This suggests that although individual SNSs may rise and fall, the phenomenon of SNSs is likely to endure for the near future.

TWITTER

Twitter (www.twitter.com) began in 2006 as a site focused on microblogging. Users are able to post *tweets*, 140-character posts, about recent events, ideas, or even random thoughts. In addition to generating their own tweets, Twitter users can choose to *follow* the Twitter posts of other Twitter users. Twitter followers are then notified of and can view every tweet that is generated by the person being followed. As of 2011, Twitter was the ninth most popular Web site in the world.[9] In contrast to Myspace and

Facebook, the majority of members on Twitter are adults. The 2009 study of 1828 high school students using SNSs found that only 0.2% used Twitter, and slightly less than 1% of 1174 college students preferred Twitter to other SNSs.[8] Recent Twitter feeds by famous actors and singers, however, have gained popularity among adolescents, as demonstrated by the 12 million followers of Lady Gaga on Twitter.

Given the popularity of these sites and the amount of time adolescents spend using them, it seems reasonable to ask the question, "What impact do SNSs have on adolescents' health and well-being?" There has been increasing research in the past decade toward understanding the risks of SNS use, with topics ranging from older fears, such as adult Internet predators and social withdrawal, to new unique concerns, such as cyberbullying and sexting. Benefits to SNS use have also been better understood and defined. More recently, research has provided insights on the benefits and risks to pediatricians of SNSs.

RISKS TO ADOLESCENTS
Displayed Health Risk Behaviors

Many of the major causes of morbidity and mortality in US adolescents are related to risky health behaviors, such as violence, sexual activity, and substance use.[10] Because SNSs, such as Facebook, give adolescents the opportunity to post information about their personal lives, such as likes, dislikes, and activities, they also present an opportunity for adolescents to display information about risky behaviors, both in text and picture format. These displays are not uncommon; previous research has shown that approximately half of all adolescent SNS profiles contain references to risky health behaviors. A study of older adolescents on Myspace found that 41% of SNS profiles referenced substance use, 24% referenced sex, and 14% referenced violent behavior.[3] There are two ways in which these public displays referencing risk behaviors may present risks to adolescents.

First, many adolescents do not realize that even with privacy settings available on SNSs, once information is posted online, it is often permanent and available for others to view. A previous study found that 75% of adolescents were unaware that online content that has been uploaded cannot be permanently deleted.[11] Future employers, school admissions panels, and other adult role models may be able to view and make judgments based on displayed online information.

A second risk to the public display of health risk behaviors on SNSs is the potential influence these displays could have on other, particularly younger, adolescents. Studies have shown that adolescents often believe SNS references to be accurate, which may influence their own perceptions and actions. It has been postulated that SNSs act as a "superpeer," combining the influence of traditional media with the power of interpersonal persuasion.[3] It is possible that when adolescents view comments about sexual activity or substance use on another user's profile that did not result in any negative consequences, this could be a powerful tool of persuasion that results in engagement of those same activities by other adolescents. In addition to influencing the behavior of others, posting information about risky health behaviors may influence others' opinions about the person displaying the information. For example, using focus groups, Moreno and colleagues[12] found that displayed sexual references on female college students SNS profiles increased the sexual expectations of college men.

Cyberbullying

Cyberbullying is defined as the deliberate use of social media to communicate false, embarrassing, or hostile information about another individual.[13] It can include name calling, spreading rumors, pretending to be someone else, sending unwanted pictures or texts, distributing pictures without consent, making threats, or asking someone to do something sexual.[11] Although cyberbullying can have similar consequences as traditional offline bullying, such as depression and anxiety, there are some unique aspects of cyberbullying that may increase the potential severity of these consequences. For instance, because it occurs online, cyberbullying can occur at any time, not just when face to face.[11] Additionally, given the wide use of SNSs, cyberbullying has the potential to reach a large audience, which can increase the embarrassment factor.[11]

Estimates of the prevalence of cyberbullying range from 6% to 42% in the United States.[14] This large range is likely due to the lack of a standardized definition of cyberbullying; studies that used narrow definitions of behaviors found more narrow ranges of estimates of the behavior. For example, a study of middle school students found that 29.5% of boys and 27.8% of girls have posted a "rude or nasty" comment on an SNS page.[8] Although there are concerns that cyberbullying is a more anonymous form of bullying, one study found that 73% of youth knew the identity of the cyberbully.[11]

It is unclear if the prevalence of cyberbullying varies by gender. One study found that boys were more likely than girls to be perpetrators and girls more likely than boys to be victims of cyberbullying.[14] Another study, however, demonstrated no differences between genders in regards to perpetrators of cyberbullying, although it did find that older female adolescents (10th and 11th graders) were more likely to be victims of cyberbullying than male adolescents of the same age.[11] Despite these unknowns, cyberbullying can have significant psychosocial effects on the victims, including depression, anxiety, social isolation, and even suicide attempts. Several headline cases of suicide in the media have raised awareness and concern about these consequences.

Sexting

The term, *sexting*, refers to sending, receiving, or forwarding sexually explicit messages or pictures over cell phones, computers, or other digital devices.[13] A recent survey found that 20% of teens have sent or posted nude or seminude photos or videos of themselves.[13] In most cases these photos were intended to be viewed only by a boyfriend or girlfriend. A survey in 2008 revealed, however, that 40% of teens and young adults had been shown a message of a sexual nature that had been intended for someone else.[8] In recent years, there have been news reports about adolescents who have been charged with felony child pornography or juvenile law misdemeanors as a result of sexting messages that reached beyond the intended audience.[13] Other consequences of sexting include emotional distress and school suspensions.

Online Solicitation

Given the anonymity of the Internet and the ease with which identity can be disguised, concerns have been raised about child predators using SNSs to solicit adolescents. A study assessing the online patterns of sexual offenders (both Internet and non-Internet offenders) performed from 2008 to 2009 found that 74.5% of past offenders were unwilling to answer questions about their use of SNSs, even though "none used" was an option.[8] In this same study, those past offenders who did admit to using SNSs named Myspace as the most commonly visited site.[8] Additionally, more than half of the Internet offenders admitted to disguising their identity while online, and

63.3% reported that they initiated conversations about sexual activity during their first contact with a stranger online.[8]

Although a study done in 2008 demonstrated that youth were less likely to be solicited on an SNS compared with in a chat room, the danger is present and measurable.[2] A national survey of 10 to 15 year olds who had used the Internet within the preceding 6 months found that 15% had experienced an unwanted sexual solicitation while online within the past year.[15] Despite concerns about adults soliciting adolescents for sexual activities, however, most recent studies found that sexual solicitation most often occurs between two teenagers instead of between teenagers and adults.

BENEFITS TO ADOLESCENTS FROM SNSs

Not all the research on SNSs, however, is concerning. Many studies in recent years have emphasized the potential benefits SNSs can have for adolescents.

Mental Health and Development

Ask just about any parent of a teenager: adolescence can be a time of high drama, insecurities, and frequent mood swings. The mental health of adolescents is a heavily researched concept; it is unsurprising, then, that the effect of SNSs on adolescent mental health has attracted the attention of researchers.

In 2006, Dutch researchers found that adolescents who had experienced a greater number of positive reactions to their SNS profile also experienced higher self-esteem and satisfaction with their life.[2] Comparably, in 2009, a study of college students in Texas demonstrated that Facebook usage was positively correlated with life satisfaction, social trust, and civic engagement.[2] Epidemiologic studies over the years have repeatedly demonstrated that as the size of users' social networks increase, so does their overall health.[16] There may be a limit in social network size for this benefit, because research suggests that those with extremely large social networks may have a decrease in the quality of their interactions with others, with superficial engagement substituting for meaningful relationships.[16]

Along with surviving the drama of adolescence, one of the most important milestones in adolescence is the development of an identity, a sense of self with experiences, morals, and beliefs that help guide future decisions. SNSs give adolescents opportunities to explore and shape their identity by choosing what information about themselves to display to the public and how the information they display changes in response to new experiences as well as how it relates to feedback from peers. Additionally, for those adolescents with interests outside the mainstream culture, SNSs provide an outlet for meeting new people with shared interests. These online peer groups may provide adolescents with the support they need to develop an identity that they may not have been able to do offline.[3]

Education and Civic Engagement

At first glance, it may seem strange that Facebook and other SNSs could have any positive effect on education, considering that time spent with social media is time spent not doing homework. Initial studies suggested a correlation between increased usage of Facebook and lower grade point average, contributing to many schools blocking SNSs from being accessible on the schools' Internet networks.[2] Recent studies have not found any relationship (either positive or negative) between SNS usage and grade point average, however.[2] Additionally, there are many reports of teachers and schools using SNSs as teaching tools to improve interest and adolescent engagement in academic activities. John Chase, a teacher in New York, has created online and multimedia assignments for students that often address topics that are challenging to teach in traditional formats. Examples include assignments designed to improve understanding of dyslexia and those contemplating bullying and suicide (http://www.classroom20.com/profile/JohnathanChase). A common use of SNSs in schools is blogging to help increase skills in creative writing.[2,13]

In addition to directly using SNSs in classroom assignments, these sites can be used as a means of communication between students as well as between students and teachers to discuss homework assignments and projects.[13] These online tools allow for easy collaboration while eliminating the hassle of arranging and organizing meeting times outside of school.

Because of the ease of communicating quickly with large groups of people, SNSs are tools not only for finding help on homework assignments but also for organizing large group events. One feature of SNSs, such as Facebook, is the ability to create groups and events, which can be private or publicly available to others on the site. Many of the existing groups on Facebook are dedicated to political, religious, or community purposes, allowing adolescents to meet people and discuss ideas with others. A national survey of 1000 adolescents and young adults ages 14 to 22 found that those who used the Internet more often were more politically aware and civically engaged compared with those who used the Internet less often.[17] In recent years, there have been anecdotal reports of adolescents using SNSs to organize beneficial activities, ranging from church outings to political campaigns.[3]

Social Capital

The term, *social capital*, is used in many different ways, with a wide range of definitions. All of these definitions are based on the idea that social networks have value and that individuals can derive benefit from their interactions and relationships with others.[2] Given that SNSs allow individuals to create larger social networks than they could offline, it seems logical that using an SNS could help adolescents build social capital. A study in 2007 found that increased Facebook use was positively correlated with bridging and bonding social capital in college students.[2]

There are several hypothesized ways in which online social networks could bring benefit to adolescents. For instance, SNSs allow adolescents to access health information that they may be too uncomfortable to ask a pediatrician about, and they also allow adolescents with a chronic disease to join online support groups to help them deal with new diagnoses or share stories with others who understand their situation in life.[13] Additionally, SNSs give adolescents the benefit of being able to start and maintain relationships despite physical distance.[18]

THE ROLE OF PEDIATRICIANS REGARDING SNSs

It is challenging to dispute the important role that SNSs and other technologies play in the lives of adolescents, and previous research has shown that SNSs can have both positive and negative impacts on adolescents. Thus, it is reasonable that every pediatrician should have at least a basic understanding of SNSs and be comfortable discussing the risks and benefits of these sites with adolescents and parents. Research suggests, however, that only 3.6% of clinicians routinely counsel their patients about Internet use and 33.3% of clinicians have never discussed the Internet with their patients, although American Academy of Pediatrics recommendations include asking a minimum of two media questions at every well child visit. Some pediatricians may argue they lack training or adequate knowledge about SNSs and the Internet to counsel families. Other pediatricians suggest that there is an obligation to learn about topics that have significant effects on children and adolescent lives. Toward this goal, the American Academy of Pediatrics provides expert advice and recommendations for education about the Internet and media safety that physicians can use as a tool for discussion with adolescents and parents. Even a pediatrician without much working knowledge of SNSs and the Internet can encourage parents to take a more active role in monitoring their children's online activities and remind teenagers that once something is posted online, it is difficult, if not impossible, to permanently remove.[13] Studies have shown that teenagers who are directly warned about inappropriate content in their online profiles are more likely than others to make changes in the content and privacy settings.[4]

Pediatricians are in a unique role to educate patients and families about the risks and benefits to adolescents from SNSs.[13] Are there other incentives, however, besides patient education to encourage pediatricians to learn about SNSs? Recent research has focused on this question and whether or not there are direct benefits and risks to pediatricians from SNSs.

Risks to Pediatricians from SNSs

Given that the newest generation of physicians grew up in the era of technology, many young residents, fellows, and physicians have their own profiles on SNSs. A study in 2010 found that 88% of providers in the study had a personal SNS account, although trainees were more likely to have a profile than faculty.[18] Likewise, a 2009 study in France found that 73% of residents and fellows had a Facebook profile.[19] This large percentage of young physicians who actively use SNSs has led to discussions about professionalism and Health Insurance Portability and Accountability Act (HIPAA) regulations in the age of social media.

Professionalism

Epstein and Hundert define professionalism as "the habitual and judicious use of communication, knowledge, technical skills, clinical reasoning, emotions, values, and reflection in daily practice for the benefit of the individual and community being served."[20] The Accreditation Council for Graduate Medical Education states that every physician should demonstrate "professional accountability to society,"[21] and in 2002 the Medical Professionalism Project launched a professionalism charter that included 10 professional responsibilities, including commitments to professional competence, honesty with patients, patient confidentiality, maintaining appropriate relations with patients, improving quality of care, improving access to care, a just distribution of finite resources, scientific knowledge, maintaining trust by managing conflicts of interest, and professional responsibilities.[22]

Perhaps never before has the line between a physician's work persona and personal persona been as blurred as it is now in the age of social media. For those physicians who maintain an SNS profile, personal information about themselves that would never have been revealed in an office or hospital setting may now be readily accessible to patients and their families via the Internet. A study at the University of Florida in 2008 found that of the 44.5% of residents and medical students who owned an SNS profile and two-thirds had a public profile with no privacy settings.[23]

It is worth considering whether certain personal information on a physician's profile could affect the level of trust that a patient places in the provider, thus undermining the patient-doctor relationship. For instance, the sharing of political and religious beliefs on a profile page may affect how much information a patient decides to disclose for fear of judgment.[24]

The most heavily researched area involves the display of unprofessional behaviors, either by text or pictures, on a provider's SNS profiles. Several studies have shown that the most frequent unprofessional behaviors displayed on SNS profiles of medical professionals include alcohol use and offensive language.[24] These displays can take the form of text references or pictures of substance use or use of sexist or racist language or text that shows a lack of respect for a patient.[23] In the study at the University of Florida in 2008, 70% of resident and medical student profiles included at least one picture of the individual consuming alcohol, and up to 50% of the pictures demonstrated excessive drinking.[23] These displays are especially detrimental to pediatricians working with adolescents and young adults, because displays of substance use or drinking could have a negative impact on a physician's credibility when counseling patients about drinking and other risky health behaviors.

In addition to displaying unprofessional behavior and language, physicians who recount stories about their professional lives on SNSs also risk violating HIPAA regulations and their professional commitment to maintaining patient confidentiality. Even when physicians attempt to edit out names to protect patients, they may inadvertently include enough details that patients can be identified.[24]

Is friending a patient appropriate?
A major factor in the quality of health care that a patient receives is the quality of the patient-doctor relationship. This may be especially true for pediatricians who work with adolescents. Trust, mutual respect, and a nonjudgmental attitude are essential for developing a rapport with adolescents, which in turn can lead to openness and full disclosure about possible risky health behaviors. Also important to the patient-doctor relationship with adolescents is connecting with them on their level. In recent years, pediatricians have begun corresponding with their adolescent patients via e-mail in an attempt to increase access and communication with physicians. Recent data suggest, however, that many teens prefer using Facebook messaging to communicating with traditional e-mail.[3] This practice raises several questions. To communicate via Facebook, should pediatricians become "friends" with their patients, thus allowing these adolescents access to personal information about pediatricians? If so, how does friending between pediatricians and adolescents affect the patient-doctor relationship?

The study performed in France in 2009 found that 6% of participating residents and fellows had received a friend request from a patient, and 50% of these accepted the friend request.[19] The investigators then asked the remaining 94% of residents and fellows who had not received a friend request how they would react if the situation presented itself. Nearly all residents and fellows (85%) stated they would automatically decline the friend request, citing reasons, such as needing to keep a distance between themselves and their patients, wishing to protect their own personal information, considering the interaction unethical, or suspecting the patient of wanting a romantic relationship.[19] Almost half of participants believed the patient-doctor relationship would change even if the patient just knew the pediatrician had a Facebook profile, and 76% believed the relationship would be significantly altered if the patient had access to the provider's profile information.[19] The remaining 15% who would not automatically decline the request stated they would decide on an individual basis. Reasons given for possibly accepting a friend request included feeling a special affinity with a patient, fear of embarrassing a patient, fear of losing a patient, or fear of losing a patient's confidence.[19]

Screening candidates
Building rapport and trust with adolescents is a difficult task for many pediatricians. It is easy to see how it could be tempting for a pediatrician to look up a patient's

Facebook profile to gather more information about a patient. Another motivator may be to seek information about substance use or risky sexual behaviors, because adolescents often post references to these behaviors. So the question arises, is it ethical to look up information about a patient on SNSs, and, if so, what should be done with the information obtained?

One survey found that trainees and faculty, in general, believed it was not an invasion of privacy to conduct Internet or SNS searches of patients, as long as they do not have special privacy settings.[18] In addition, a study of 302 psychotherapy graduate students found that 27% had sought information about a patient from an SNS, for reasons ranging from curiosity to establishing the truth to gathering more background information.[18] Other studies, however, show that adolescents and physicians tend to have different perceptions about whether content on SNSs is considered public versus private, with many adolescents feeling it is a violation of privacy to have physicians search their SNS profiles for health behaviors.[18]

The second question about what to do with the information obtained is likely more complicated than whether or not to look for the information in the first place. For instance, if an adolescent denies alcohol use in clinic, but a physician discovers pictures of the patient drinking on Facebook, should the physician confront the patient with this information? Alternatively disclosing that the physician is aware of the patient's drinking could lead the adolescent to feeling as though his or her privacy was violated, potentially having an impact on the patient-doctor relationship and reducing any chance of future trust. By ignoring the evidence, however, the physician is denied an opportunity for counseling or education, and the patient could suffer serious health consequences from alcohol use. In an even more serious situation, if during a search of a patient's SNS profile, a physician uncovers evidence that a patient has been a victim of abuse or violence or is having suicidal thoughts, is this sufficient evidence of suspicion for the physician to conduct mandatory reporting? Anecdotal evidence suggests that in these cases, contacting the patient or an appropriate authority to determine the validity of this information is supported by physicians' roles as mandatory reporters for suspicion of harm or abuse.

Benefits to Pediatricians from SNSs

Although there are sufficient data on the risks of SNSs for pediatricians, there is little research on the direct benefits of SNSs for pediatricians. A few studies have investigated how SNSs can be beneficial to health care organizations and providers in general and other studies postulate potential benefits to pediatricians.

Promoting practice

Social media has the ability to reach large masses of people, and as such, is ideal for promoting practices and services that are available. As of July 2010, 762 health care organizations maintained some sort of social media presence for various reasons, such as customer service, community outreach, patient education, public relations, and crisis communications.[25] Twitter seemed the most common SNS used by health care organizations, with 583 hospitals maintaining a Twitter account.[25] Second-most popular was Facebook, with 551 hospitals maintaining a profile page.[25]

A review of Facebook profiles from several pediatric hospitals in the Midwestern United States revealed that most of these pages contained information about the hospital, including size, location, contact information, and maps. Additionally, most profiles included a *wall*, where information about upcoming events is posted as well as comments from satisfied patients and families. Most profiles contained miniblog entries about various pediatric health topics from hospital providers. Some profiles had special sections about donation opportunities, special recipes for children, and pictures of patients who had received care at that institution.[6]

Patient and family education

A unique benefit of SNSs is that they are able to reach vast audiences in minimal time. This makes SNSs a potentially effective tool for distributing health care information to patients and families. The World Health Organization used Twitter during the H1N1 influenza pandemic to give updates about severity, availability of vaccine, and other information to 11,700 followers.[26] Additionally, the Centers for Disease Control and prevention maintains a Twitter account that boasts 420,000 followers.[26] Many surgeons have also taken to tweeting in the operating room as an educational tool to help alleviate fears before surgery by promoting transparency in health care and demystifying the inner workings of an operating room.[27]

Another unique example of using an SNS for health education is the Seattle Mama Doc blog (seattlemamadoc.seattlechildrens.org). Dr Wendy Sue Swanson, a pediatrician from Seattle Children's Hospital, maintains a blog and Twitter account to write about various pediatric health care topics, ranging from infant development to vaccinations to safety to obesity to teenage health concerns. She not only writes articles from her own perspective but also frequently invites colleagues to be guest bloggers about important topics. Additionally, she often posts new pediatric research articles and then deciphers the findings into family-friendly language.[28]

Improved interactions with teens

Several articles have suggested that SNSs could be used to improve interactions with adolescents, as a way to meet them on their own turf, so to speak. Several studies have suggested that adolescents prefer communicating via SNSs as opposed to traditional e-mail.[3] Additionally, most adolescents have cell phone access, making text messaging a new, interesting route for communication with pediatricians. For example, there have been some initial investigations into the use of text messaging and SNSs to help newly diagnosed diabetic adolescents manage their disease.[29]

Another idea regarding how SNSs may be used to interact with adolescents is the use of Facebook profile pages in a clinical office setting. Some have proposed looking over a patient's profile page with the patient, as a novel way to take a social history.[3] There are no research studies to date on how this would work in a clinical setting or how physicians might carve out time in a busy clinic schedule to pursue such activities.

SUMMARY

Given the prevalence of social media and SNSs in today's world and the significant role they play in the lives of adolescents, it is advisable that every pediatrician be aware of the research findings regarding SNSs and adolescents. Pediatricians are in a unique role to offer education about the risks and benefits of SNSs to adolescent patients and their families and to offer advice on how to minimize the risks without decreasing the benefits. Pediatricians should also be knowledgeable about the possible impact, both positive and negative, that SNSs could have on their own professional lives. SNSs are currently an active area of research, with new risks and benefits reported frequently. Fortunately, it is a physician's job to never stop learning.

REFERENCES

1. Rideout VJ, Foehr UG, Roberts D. Generation M2: media in the lives of 8 to 18 year olds. Menlo Park (CA): Kaiser Family Foundation; 2010.

2. Ahn J. The effect of social network sites on adolescents' social and academic development: current theories and controversies. J Am Soc Inform Sci Tech 2011;62(8):1435–45.

3. Moreno MA. Social networking sites and adolescents. Pediatr Ann 2010;39(9): 565–8.

4. Patchin JW, Hinduja S. Changes in adolescent online social networking behaviors from 2006 to 2009. Comput Hum Behav 2010;26(6):1818–21.

5. Lenhart A, Madden M. Teens, privacy and online social networks. Available at: Pew Internet and American Life Project; 2007.

6. Facebook. 2011. Available at: www.facebook.com. Accessed March 16, 2012.

7. Childs M. Facebook surpasses Google in weekly US hits for first time. Business week; 2010.

8. Dowdell EB, Burgess AW, Flores JR. Online social networking patterns among adolescents, young adults, and sexual offenders. Am J Nurs 2011;111(7):28–36.

9. Alexa: The Web Information Company. Alexa Internet Inc, 2011. Available at: www.alexa.com(http://www.alexa.com/). Accessed March 16, 2012.

10. Neinstein L, Anderson M. Adolescent development. In: Neinstein L, editor. Adolescent health care: a practical guide. Philadelphia: Lippincott Williams and Wilkins; 2002. p. 767–92.

11. Mishna F, Cook C, Gadalla T, et al. Cyber bullying behaviors among middle and high school students. Am J Orthopsychiatry 2010;80:362–74.

12. Moreno MA, Swanson MJ, Royer H, et al. Sexpectations: male college students' views about displayed sexual references on females' social networking web sites. J Pediatr Adolesc Gynecol 2011;24(2):85–9.

13. O'Keeffe GS, Clarke-Pearson K. Clinical report—the impact of social media on children, adolescents, and families. Pediatrics 2011;127(4):800–4.

14. Wang J, Iannotti RJ, Nansel TR. School bullying among adolescents in the United States: physical, verbal, relational, and cyber. J Adolesc Health 2009;45:368–75.

15. Ybarra ML, Espelage DL, Mitchell KJ. The co-occurrence of Internet harassment and unwanted sexual solicitation victimization and perpetration: associations with psychosocial indicators. J Adolesc Health 2007;41:S31–41.

16. Rajani R, Berman DS, Rozanski A. Social networks—are they good for your health? The era of Facebook and Twitter. QJM 2011;104:819–20.

17. Jackson LA. Adolescents and the Internet. In: Romer D, Jamieson P, editors. The Changing Portrayal of American Youth in Popular Media. Pennsylvania (NY): Oxford University Press; 2008. p. 377–410.

18. Jent JF, Eaton CK, Merrick MT, et al. The decision to access patient information from a social media site: what would you do? J Adolesc Health 2011;49(4):414–20.

19. Moubarak G, Guiot A, Benhamou Y, et al. Facebook activity of residents and fellows and its impact on the doctor-patient relationship. J Med Ethics 2011;37: 101–4.

20. Epstein RM, Hundert EM. Defining and assessing professional competence. JAMA 2002;287(2):226–35.

21. ACME Competencies: Common Program Requirements. ACGME 2008. Available at: http://www.acgme.org/acWebsite/navPages/commonpr_documents/IVA5e_EducationalProgram_ACGMECompetencies_Professionalism_Explanation.pdf. Accessed March 16, 2012.

22. Kirk LM. Professionalism in medicine: definitions and considerations for teaching. Proc (Bayl Univ Med Cent) 2007;20(1):13–6.

23. Thompson LA, Dawson K, Ferdig R, et al. The intersection of online social networking with medical professionalism. J Gen Intern Med 2008;23(7):954–7.

24. MacDonald J, Sohn S, Ellis P. Privacy, professionalism and Facebook: a dilemma for young doctors. Med Educ 2010;44:805–13.
25. Eckler P, Worsowicz G, Rayburn JW. Social media and health care: an overview. PM R 2010;2(11):1046–50.
26. McNab C. What social media offers to health professionals and citizens. Bull World Health Organ 2009;87(8):566.
27. Coffield RL, Joiner JE. Risky Business: treating tweeting the symptoms of social media. AHLA Connections 2010;14(3):10–4.
28. Swanson, WS. Seattle Mama Doc 2011. Available at: www.seattlemamadoc. seattlechildrens.org(http://www.seattlemamadoc.seattlechildrens.org/). Accessed March 16, 2012.
29. Franklin VL, Greene A, Waller A, et al. Patients' engagement with "Sweet Talk"— a text messaging support system for young people with diabetes. J Med Internet Res 2008;10(2):e20.

Should Babies Be Watching Television and DVDs?

Ellen A. Wartella, PhD*, Alexis R. Lauricella, PhD

KEYWORDS

- DVD • Developmental outcomes • Hypotheses • Infants • Learning • TV
- Video deficit

KEY POINTS

- Infants and toddlers are regular viewers of television and DVD content.
- Research related to infant media use is increasing but evidence is mixed.
- It is important for infants to learn how to watch and learn from screen media.

SHOULD BABIES BE WATCHING TELEVISION/DVDs?

It has been 15 years since the first *Baby Einstein* video came on the market. Since 1997, there has been a proliferation of a variety of screen media developed for babies (eg, DVDs, cable television channels, Web sites, apps, e-books).[1] Marketing campaigns for infant-directed products have insinuated that children learn from DVDs like *Baby Einstein* and *Brainy Baby*, convincing many parents that these products are educational. On the other hand, the American Academy of Pediatrics (AAP) originally recommended that parents "avoid TV- and video-viewing for children less than age 2"[2] and more recently the AAP[3] "discourages media use by children younger than 2 years." These conflicting messages, along with the proliferation of digital technology in our daily lives, makes the question of whether babies should be watching television and DVDs a reasonable one to ask but a difficult one to answer.

First, regardless of these conflicting messages, infants and toddlers are watching television and DVDs, and many children were watching even before the boom of infant-directed media.[4] According to parental reports of media use in the early 1990s, 1-year-old infants watched an hour of television on an average day.[5] More recent media use studies have noted that babies are watching television more regularly than before.[6] For 1-year-olds, about half watched television in the mid-1990s compared with 60% in 2003.[6] In 2006, the Kaiser Family Foundation survey[7] found

Communication Studies, Northwestern University, 2-148 Frances Searle Building, 2240 Campus Drive, Evanston, IL 60208, USA
* Corresponding author.
E-mail address: ewartella@gmail.com

Pediatr Clin N Am 59 (2012) 613–621
doi:10.1016/j.pcl.2012.03.027   pediatric.theclinics.com
0031-3955/12/$ – see front matter © 2012 Elsevier Inc. All rights reserved.

that children younger than 1 year spent on average just less than an hour a day (49 minutes) with screen media. According to the most recent Common Sense Media survey,[8] 66% of children younger than 2 years have watched television and almost half watch television or DVDs in a typical day. Children younger than 2 years who did watch television spent about 1 hour a day watching television, which is consistent with the amount of time infants were watching in the late 1970s.[9]

Second, although total amount of time children are watching television and DVDs is important, past research with older children shows that the content they are watching on television is also crucial.[10,11] A national representative survey of parents found that most children (83%) watched programming that was created for children around their own age.[7] Parents of children younger than 2 years reported that their children mostly watched programming for children, but 19% of parents reported that their children watched a mix of programming for both children and adults.[7] The most recent nationally representative survey did not report the specific types of television and video content that very young children were watching,[8] so it is unclear what content young infants and babies are currently watching on television.

Television is ubiquitous in American homes, and babies are attending to television and videos, especially to the growing number of media products developed for them. As a result, scientists and researchers have begun to research infants' media use. Rather than examining the literature to explore evidence that is for or against early television viewing, here we explore the current hypotheses and evidence about infants' media use at home more generally.

Attention Hypotheses

Historically, there were 2 theories regarding children's attention to television. Anderson and colleagues[12] theorized that attention was driven by the comprehensibility of the content, known as the comprehensibility hypothesis, whereas Huston and Wright[13] theorized that formal features that occur on television, such as auditory and visual changes, drive attention, which became known as the formal features hypothesis. Both of these theories were originally based on the understanding of preschool-aged children's viewing of television programming but have been applied to the understanding of infant and toddlers' attention to television programming as well.

Comprehensibility hypothesis

Anderson and colleagues[12] discovered in the early 1980s that young children's (ages 2, 3.5, and 5 years) attention to television was driven by the comprehensibility of the content, meaning that if children understood the content they attended more. In the new century, Pempek and colleagues[14] applied this same theory and tested it on a younger audience of infants younger than 24 months. Evidence from this study found that infants as young as 18 months old are sensitive to changes in comprehensibility of programming. For example, 18-month-old and 24-month-old infants attended less to segments of *Teletubbies* that had been edited to decrease their comprehensibility (random shot sequences and backward speech) than those that were not distorted.[14]

Formal features hypothesis

An early study by Hollenbeck and Slaby[9] found infants' attention was highest when they watched a traditional type of television program that included both sound and picture compared with either sound-only or picture-only experiences. More recently, Valkenburg and Vroone[15] found that infants' attention was attracted to the screen when there were salient auditory and visual features, such as applause, a child's voice, bright colors, or visual surprises on the screen. These studies have examined infants' attention to formal features but did not specifically test the formal features hypothesis. Other research has begun to examine the extent of formal production features used in infant-directed videos,[16] but again this study did not examine infant attention to these various types of formal features.

Developmental Outcomes Hypothesis

Historically, new technology and change in family routines bring concerns about the possible harmful consequences.[17] When television and video programs were first created and marketed directly for infants and toddlers, concerns about the impact of such early exposure were ignited. In response to the creation of infant-directed products and reports that infants and toddlers were watching television, the AAP issued a policy statement in 1999[2] recommending that parents avoid television viewing for children younger than 2 years. As part of this recommendation, the AAP stated that "there is concern that overstimulation from high levels of media use might lead to attention deficit disorder or hyperactivity." As a result, there has been a hypothesis that early media exposure is associated with longer-term developmental outcomes such as attention and other cognitive deficiencies.

Evidence for this hypothesis is mixed. One of the first scientific studies to be released about the effects of early media exposure claimed to find an association between early television viewing and later attention problems for children.[5] This study quickly gained attention in the popular press, causing concerns that exposure to television at early ages might lead to attention problems later in childhood. However, a reanalysis of the same national longitudinal data set identified major flaws in the original analyses of the study.[18] Foster and Watkins suggested that Christakis and colleagues[5] failed to include adequate control variables in their original analysis of the data. When Foster and Watkins included mother's academic achievement and family's poverty status as control variables in their regression analysis, the association between television viewing and attention problems was no longer statistically significant. Overall, Foster and Watkins state "modest levels of television viewing do not appear to be detrimental, even for young children".[18(p374)] A study by researchers in Denmark[19] also found no association between early television viewing (ages 8 months and 3½ years) and behavior problems related to attention-deficit/hyperactivity disorder at age 10 and 11 years old.

Multiple studies have examined language development as a function of early media exposure. Zimmerman and colleagues[20] found that viewing DVDs created for infants between 8 and 16 months of age was associated with worse concurrent language scores on the Communicative Development Inventory (CDI). Exposure for older toddlers (17–24 months) was not associated with CDI language scores. In contrast, a longitudinal study of infants from age 6 months to 3 years showed that when a range of other demographic variables were controlled for, there was no association between hours of early television viewing and language scores as measured by the Peabody Picture Vocabulary Test at age 3 years.[21] In addition, smaller-scale studies indicate no association between early television and video viewing and language or other cognitive outcomes. Specifically, language scores as measured by the CDI were not significantly predicted by the DVD viewing frequency of infants.[22]

In addition to frequency of viewing, studies have examined the potential influence of media content on later outcomes. A small study found that language development varied based on the specific educational programs children watched before age 2 years.[23] The importance of content was evident in a low-risk sample: early exposure to infant-directed programming had no association with later cognitive, school readiness, or executive functioning skills; however, exposure to content created for adults at early ages was associated with worse executive function skills.[24]

Educational Hypotheses

The proven success of planned educational programs such as *Sesame Street* to teach preschool-aged children language and mathematical concepts gave rise to an explosion of preschool television, video, and digital products claiming to be educational for children.[1] However, even with substantial evidence that preschoolers could learn from video, early on researchers were skeptical that television and DVD products could be educational for younger children, specifically infants and toddlers. This skepticism was reinforced by evidence of a video deficit in baby's learning from video[6] and only recently has evidence shown that although there may be constraints on babies learning from video, such learning can and may occur under certain circumstances. Richert and colleagues[25] recently suggested that the challenges that infants face when learning from screen media may be a result of their lack of understanding of the social significance of screen media. More specifically, infants need to learn that what they view on a screen can provide them with information about their world and can be a tool for learning.[25]

Video deficit hypothesis

Initial research of infant and toddler media found that infants and toddlers learn better from a real-world adult than they do from a video presentation, thus coining the term the video deficit.[6] Evidence in support of this hypothesis has been shown in a range of experimental studies until infants are between 2 and 3 years old.[26–28] Imitation studies conducted with infants from 12 to 30 months old have shown that learning of a 1-step to 3-step imitation task is significantly better when the infant views the demonstration performed live by an adult compared with the same demonstration performed on a screen.[29,30] Similar evidence has been found using object-search tasks, showing that toddlers are better able to find hidden objects when information about their hiding places is provided by a live adult compared with when it is given on screen.[27,31–34] Evidence also shows that infants and toddlers learn language skills better from a live experience than from a video or televised presentation.[22,35,36] Together this evidence does support the theory that there is a video deficit effect for infants and toddlers and that infants may view characters on a screen differently than they view people in live interactions.[22]

However, there is also evidence that under certain circumstances this video deficit effect can be ameliorated or may even fail to exist for some audiences. First, repetition of the video presentation helped to increase learning and ameliorate the video deficit effect with 12-month-old and 18-month-old infants.[37] For 15-month-old infants, increasing the repetition of the video and spreading the exposures over 2 days ameliorated the video deficit effect.[37] In addition, with object-search tasks, young children who had 2 weeks of exposure on their home television screen before testing were better able to use a video presentation as information to successfully find a hidden toy.[34] When the test task is changed and infants are tested on their ability to learn a task from a two-dimensional (2D) screen and replicate it on a 2D touch screen, infants show learning and do not show the video deficit effect.[38] Research also shows that the video deficit effect may not occur for very young infants. For instance, 6-month-old infants learned as well from a video as from a live demonstration.[39,40]

Learning hypothesis

Decades of research with preschool-aged children have shown that educational media have benefits for preschoolers' development of literacy, mathematics, science, and prosocial behavior.[41–43] Given that older children can learn from quality educational media and marketers push products as educational,[1] it has been hypothesized that infant-directed media may be educational for infants and toddlers as well.

Since the creation of infant-directed media in the late 1990s, studies have begun to examine the ways in which infants and toddlers may learn from commercially produced and experimentally created video presentations. Infants can learn a cognitively meaningful seriation task (ordering objects according to size) better from a video presentation when the character on the screen is familiar compared with when the character is unfamiliar.[44] In addition, infants can learn to successfully complete an object-search task when they are given training and experience using screens as a source of information. For example, children who engaged with an adult on a closed-circuit television were better able to find a hidden object than children in the control group who did not experience the interactive television condition.[45,46] In addition, by providing toddlers with training experiences at home where they saw themselves on a television screen, they were then able to learn from a video presentation when they came to a laboratory to complete the object-search task.[34]

Other studies have shown that 2-year-olds can learn from video presentations even when tested 24 hours after exposure.[26,28] Toddlers in the Barr and Wyss study[26] successfully imitated the behaviors shown on video when the video contained a voice-over that provided labels during the demonstration. There is some evidence that infants may be able to learn language from programs created for them. An experimentally controlled study showed that infants who were exposed to *Baby Einstein* around age 1 year showed greater learning of specific words from the DVD compared with children in the control group who did not view the video.[47] In contrast, other studies examining infants' language learning from commercially created infant-directed videos have failed to find learning gains.[22,35,48] Thus, it is possible that infants and toddlers develop the skills necessary to comprehend and learn from television as they get older either because of increased experience or practice watching television or as a function of cognitive development factors.

Scaffolding hypothesis

According to Vygotsky's theory,[49] social interaction plays a key role in children's cognitive development. Specifically, Vygotsky focuses on the important role an adult can play by scaffolding an experience for a child, meaning that the adult can provide help and support through verbal interactions and directions to engage the child in the experience to increase learning. Considerable research has examined the positive role of parent interaction and scaffolding on joint book reading with young children, and the hypothesis that parent interaction could also support learning from a television program has been suggested and studied as well.[50]

Studies have shown that infants' attention to television increases with previous exposure and with increased parental interaction.[51] Specifically, when parents treated the on-screen images as something with relevant information for the child and identified this relevant information by asking on-topic questions or labeling, infants were more likely to interact with the video.[51] Similarly, word learning from a DVD was improved when parents interacted with their children during the viewing by directing the child's attention to the DVD and repeating the words from the DVD.[22] Scaffolding benefits have been shown to be equally as successful when the scaffolding is provided by an adult coviewer as when scaffolding is provided by a voice-over during the video presentation.[26] In both instances, toddlers learned to imitate the behaviors shown on a video.[26]

SUMMARY

The 15 years of research since the creation of infant-directed television and video programs has consistently shown 2 important concepts. First, parents are letting young babies watch and use media technology[8] regardless of policy statements urging caregivers to do otherwise. Second, although we have a better understanding of the ways in which infants use and learn from media than we did before, the evidence about the outcomes of early media use remains ambiguous and fails to provide conclusive evidence either for or against early media use. Rather, a review of the evidence seems to support the theory that infants must learn how to watch and how to learn from screens before successful learning or positive outcomes can be fully shown.[25,52]

As has been discussed, infants are watching television and DVDs, but they are also using interactive touch-screen technologies like iPads and smartphones.[8] The idea that screen use can be discouraged or in any way avoided seems almost impossible because of the extent to which screens are everywhere that children are: in the backseat of minivans, at supermarkets, and in their parents' hands. Not only are screens pervasive in American society, the new types of media screens are also easier for infants and toddlers to manipulate, changing the media experience from one in which infants must simply watch to one in which infants can control and interact. Similarly, a screen is no longer just a screen. Television and DVDs allow infants and toddlers to watch a previously created program that was set in length and content and created largely to provide entertainment for children. Today, screens are used for a variety of purposes including communication, information retrieval, and joint play: grandparents in Boston use Skype to see and talk to their grandchildren in Chicago; preschoolers use computers to watch YouTube videos of African lions running in the Sahara desert; and toddlers play virtual tea party with their parents on an iPad. Infants and toddlers are watching television and DVDs and are already adapting to the new technologies that are becoming a part of the culture and world in which they are developing.

The world of technology that infants are now growing up in is one that is still new. The body of evidence and our understanding about infants' media use are growing, but we are still far from having enough scientific evidence to determine whether or not infants should or should not be watching. There is evidence both for and against the two theories of attention to television, suggesting that both comprehensibility and formal features play a role in infants' attention to television and videos. There is some conflicting evidence about the cognitive deficit hypothesis that suggests that we really do not know how early media exposure influences later cognitive outcomes. There is solid evidence in favor of the video deficit effect, indicating that infants and toddlers learn better from a live experience than from one portrayed on video, but does that mean that infants cannot learn from a video presentation? The evidence suggests that there are ways in which learning can occur even at very young ages, and there is evidence that adding a live adult or scaffolding experiences can help enhance infants' chances of learning.

This review suggests that infants need to learn how to learn from screen media. Like other experiences in their lives in which they learn, for example, that blocks can teach them about physics, coins can teach them about numbers and currency, and books can teach them to read, infants, through experience and practice, need to figure out that the material that they see on a screen is a symbol of something in the real world and something that could provide them with information to learn about the world around them.

Babies' interest in television and other screen media seems to be a natural outgrowth of their interest in the objects and activities of the adults in their lives. Screens of all sorts are everywhere that adults are. The phenomena of parent's passing back smartphones to keep their children amused, or having televisions available in the family car; or joint engagement around the iPad, computer, or television are typically examined for the parental motivations for bringing media to babies. It could also be pointed out that in the process of learning about people, what motivates their actions, and how they behave, babies typically interact with the objects that occupy the adults in their lives, whether these objects are pots and pans, hats and shoes, or iPads and televisions. Screens, and most especially television, are such ubiquitous adult objects that even babies are watching.

REFERENCES

1. Garrison M, Christakis DA. A teacher in the living room? Educational media for babies, toddlers, and preschoolers. Kaiser Family Foundation; 2005.
2. Media education. American Academy of Pediatrics. Committee on Public Education. Pediatrics 1999;104:341–2.
3. Council on Communications and Media. American Academy of Pediatrics. Policy statement on media education. Pediatrics 2011;126:1–7.
4. Wartella E, Richert R, Robb M. Babies, television, and videos: how did we get here? Dev Rev 2010;30(2):116–27.
5. Christakis DA, Zimmerman FJ, DiGuiseppe DL. Early television exposure and subsequent attentional problems in children. Pediatrics 2004;113:708–13.
6. Anderson DR, Pempek TA. Television and very young children. Am Behav Sci 2005;48:505–22.
7. Rideout V, Hamel R. The media family: electronic media in the lives of infants, toddlers, preschoolers, and their parents. Menlo Park (CA): Henry J. Kaiser Family Foundation; 2006.
8. Zero to eight: children's media use in America. A common sense media research study. San Francisco (CA): Common Sense Media; 2011.
9. Hollenbeck AR, Slaby RG. Infant visual and vocal responses to television. Child Dev 1979;50:41–5.
10. Anderson DR, Huston AC, Schmitt KL, et al. Early childhood television viewing and adolescent behavior: the recontact study. Monogr Soc Res Child Dev 2001;66:I–VIII, 1–147.
11. Wright JC, Huston AC, Murphy KC, et al. The relations of early television viewing to school readiness and vocabulary of children from low-income families: the early window project. Child Dev 2001;72:1347–66.
12. Anderson DR, Lorch EP, Field DE, et al. The effect of television program comprehensibility on preschool children's visual attention to television. Child Dev 1981;52:151–7.
13. Huston AC, Wright JC. Children's processing of television: the informative functions of formal features. In: Bryant J, Anderson DR, editors. Children's understanding of television: research on attention and comprehension. New York: Academic Press; 1983. p. 35–68.
14. Pempek TA, Kirkorian HL, Richards JE, et al. Video comprehensibility and attention in very young children. Dev Psychol 2010;45:1283–93.
15. Valkenburg PM, Vroone M. Developmental changes in infants' and toddlers' attention to television entertainment. Communic Res 2004;31:288–311.
16. Goodrich S, Pempek T, Calvert SL. Formal production features in infant programming. Arch Pediatr Adolesc Med 2009;163:1151–6.
17. Wartella E, Reeves B. Historical trends in research on children and media: 1900-1960. J Commun 1985;35:118–33.
18. Foster EM, Watkins S. The value of reanalysis: TV viewing and attention problems. Child Dev 2010;81:368–75.

19. Obel C, Henriksen TB, Dalsgaard S, et al. Does children's watching of television cause attention problems? Retesting the hypothesis in a Danish cohort. Pediatrics 2004;114:1372–3.

20. Zimmerman FJ, Christakis DA, Meltzoff AN. Associations between media viewing and language development in children under 2 years. J Pediatr 2007;151:364–8.

21. Schmidt ME, Rich M, Rifas-Shiman SL, et al. Television viewing in infancy and child cognition at 3 years of age in a US cohort. Pediatrics 2009;123:e370–5.

22. Richert R, Robb M, Fender J, et al. Word learning from baby videos. Arch Pediatr Adolesc Med 2010;164:432–7.

23. Linebarger DL, Walker D. Infants' and toddlers' television viewing and language outcomes. Am Behav Sci 2005;48:624–45.

24. Barr R, Lauricella A, Zack E, et al. Infant and early childhood exposure to adult-directed and child-directed television programming. Merrill-Palmer Quarterly 2009;56:21–48.

25. Richert R, Robb MB, Smith E. Media as a social partner: the social nature of young children's learning from screen media. Child Dev 2011;82:82–95.

26. Barr R, Wyss N. Reenactment of televised content by 2-year-olds: toddlers use language learned from television to solve a difficult imitation problem. Infant Behav Dev 2008;31:696–703.

27. Schmitt KL, Anderson DR. Television and reality: toddlers' use of visual information from video to guide behavior. Media Psychol 2002;4:51–76.

28. Strouse GA, Troseth GL. "Don't try this at home": toddlers' imitation of new skills from people on video. J Exp Child Psychol 2008;101:262–80.

29. Barr R, Hayne H. Developmental changes in imitation from television during infancy. Child Dev 1999;70:1067–81.

30. Hayne H, Herbert J, Simcock G. Imitation from television by 24- and 30-months-olds. Dev Sci 2003;6:254–61.

31. Deocampo JA, Hudson JA. When seeing is not believing: two-year-olds' use of video representations to find a hidden toy. J Cognit Dev 2005;6:229–60.

32. Schmidt ME, Crawley-Davis AM, Anderson DR. Two-year-olds' object retrieval based on television: testing a perceptual account. Media Psychol 2007;9: 389–409.

33. Troseth GL, DeLoache JS. The medium can obscure the message: young children's understanding of video. Child Dev 1998;69:950–65.

34. Troseth GL. TV guide: two-year-old children learn to use video as a source of information. Dev Psychol 2003;39:140–50.

35. Kuhl PK, Tsao FM, Liu HM. Foreign-language experience in infancy: effects of short-term exposure and social interaction on phonetic learning. Proceedings of the National Academy of Sciences of the United States; 2003. p. 9096–101.

36. Naigles LR, Kako ET. First contact in verb acquisition: defining a role for syntax. Child Dev 1993;64:1665–87.

37. Barr R, Muentener P, Garcia A, et al. The effect of repetition on imitation from television during infancy. Dev Psychobiol 2007;49:196–207.

38. Zack E, Barr R, Gerhardstein P, et al. Infant imitation from television using novel touch screen technology. Br J Dev Psychol 2010;27:13–26.

39. Barr R, Muentener P, Garcia A. Age-related changes in deferred imitation from television by 6- to 18-month-olds. Dev Sci 2007;10:910–21.

40. Krcmar M. Can social meaningfulness and repeat exposure help infants and toddler overcome the video deficit. Media Psychol 2010;13:31–53.

41. Comstock G, Scharrer E. Media and the American child. Burlington (MA): Academic Press; 2007.

42. Fisch SM. Children's learning from educational television: Sesame Street and beyond. Mahwah (NJ): Lawrence Erlbaum; 2004.
43. Schmidt ME, Anderson DR. The impact of television on cognitive development and educational attainment. In: Pecora N, Murray JP, Wartella EA, editors. Children and television: fifty years of research. Mahwah (NJ): Lawrence Erlbaum Associates; 2007.
44. Lauricella AR, Gola AA, Calvert S. Toddlers' learning from socially meaningful video characters. Media Psychol 2011;14(2):216–32.
45. Nielsen M, Simcock G, Jenkins L. The effect of social engagement on 24-month-olds' imitation from live and televised models. Dev Sci 2008;11:722–31.
46. Troseth GL, Saylor MM, Archer AH. Young children's use of video as a source of socially relevant information. Child Dev 2006;77:786–99.
47. Vandewater EA. Infant world learning from commercially available video in the US. J Child Media 2011;5:248–56.
48. DeLoache JS, Choing C, Sherman K, et al. Do babies learn from baby media? Psychol Sci 2010;21:1570–4.
49. Vygotsky LS. Mind in society: the development of higher psychological processes. Cambridge (MA): Harvard University; 1978.
50. Lemish D, Rice ML. Television as a talking picture book: a prop for language acquisition. J Child Lang 1986;13:231–50.
51. Barr R, Zack E, Garcia A, et al. Attention to infant-directed programming: influence of prior exposure and parent-infant interactions. Infancy 2008;13:30–56.
52. Anderson DR. Babies and television. Beijing (China): Lecture presented at Renmin University; 2011.

Internet Bullying

Ed Donnerstein, PhD

KEYWORDS

- Internet • Cyberbullying • Aggression • Online risks • Media violence

KEY POINTS

- The era of new technology and its influence on health-related issues for children and adolescents are firmly confronting us and changing almost daily.
- These new technologies allow not only for the creation of aggression, but the ability to actually be aggressive against another, in what has been termed cyberbullying.
- The effects of being a victim of cyberbullying are often the same for youth who are bullied in person, including, for example, a drop in grades, lower self-esteem, or depression.
- In terms of solutions, the context in which online victimization occurs needs to be considered, and it is suggested that researchers examine online-related outcomes for existing evidence-based violence prevention programs.

Over the last few years, the American Academy of Pediatrics has released several Policy Statements on concerns about media violence,[1] children's advertising,[2] sexuality,[3] and other media-related health issues. The lead article in this issue by Strasburger and colleagues reviews the substantial literature on the impact of the mass media on children's and adolescents' health and development. These issues are certainly not new, but with the rapidly changing technology environment, there is an assumption that the risks to children and adolescents could be more problematic than were once expected. The question of what role new technology plays in the media's influence is now a subject of both review and discussion, particularly regarding health risks and intervention.[4,5]

The many articles in this issue address various aspects of this research. This article examines just one of these concerns, cyberbullying or Internet harassment, and considers how in a relatively short period of time a new form of acting aggressively has become part of daily conversation. In addressing this somewhat recent form of interpersonal aggression, the author takes a brief look at online usage and the theoretical mechanisms that might make Internet access more problematic in terms of risks, compared with more traditional media such as television and film. One of these risks, known today as cyberbullying (**Fig. 1**), is scrutinized in detail.

Department of Communication, University of Arizona, 1103 East University Boulevard, Tucson, AZ 85721, USA
E-mail address: edonners@u.arizona.edu

Pediatr Clin N Am 59 (2012) 623–633
doi:10.1016/j.pcl.2012.03.019
0031-3955/12/$ – see front matter © 2012 Elsevier Inc. All rights reserved.

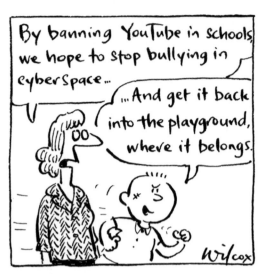

Fig. 1. Cyberbullying cartoon. (Copyright © Cathy Wilcox; reprinted with permission.)

IS ANYONE ONLINE?

The answer to this question is a simple yes. Going back to the 1960s our media platforms were television, film, radio, and the press. Eventually cable and video games were added, and concerns about these new technologies drew the attention of researchers. In looking at today's media platforms, children and adolescents now have access to the following: movies, print, radio, television, cable television, home video game consoles, portable music players, DVDs, home computers, portable handheld video game systems, Internet, cell phones, MP3 players, DVRs, electronic interactive toys, Internet-connected smart phones, tablet computers.[6] Furthermore, those few television stations of the 1960s now number in the thousands. Does this change the impact? In many ways the answer is yes.

The first question one can ask is whether these new media platforms are being used by today's youth. The answer is a definite affirmative. In their ongoing analysis of teen Internet use, the Pew Foundation[7] notes that in the last decade online use has gone from 70% to 95%, home broadband from 8% to 73%, and cell-phone use from 30% to 75% among teens (with 83% among 17-year-olds). In the last 3 years alone, smartphone use has tripled. Wireless connectivity, making the use of these new technologies easier and faster, has also shown substantial increases during this time. In its most recent study of media use, the Kaiser Foundation[8] found that Internet use among 8- to 18-year-olds has gone from 47% to 84% in the past decade, with over one-third having such access in their bedrooms. Social network sites were basically unheard of 7 years ago, yet today more than half of all Americans use a site such as Facebook (**Fig. 2**).[9]

The Kaiser study also indicated that the amount of time viewing television content had increased over the last decade, but this increase is accounted for primarily by the viewing of such programming over the Internet and mobile devices. Adolescents now spend more than 10 hours a day with some form of media. Perhaps as interesting is the Pew finding that teens actually spend more time contacting their friends via texting (54%) than through face-to-face contact (33%).[7] One should note that such findings are not restricted to the culture of American youth, being quite similar in other countries.[10,11]

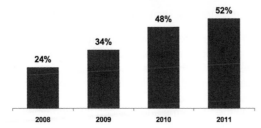

Fig. 2. Percentage of Americans who have a profile on a social networking site. (Copyright © Arbitron; reprinted with permission.)

Unlike traditional media such as television, the Internet and these new technologies (eg, mobile devices) give children and adolescents access to just about any form of content they can find. From the perspective of a child or adolescent it does not take much effort to have access to any form of violence, advertising, or sexual behavior that may be considered risky with regard to health.[4,12–15] (See article by Strasburger and colleagues elsewhere in this issue for further exploration of this topic.) Furthermore, this can be done in the privacy of their own room with little supervision from their parents.

WHAT MECHANISMS MIGHT ACCOUNT FOR NEWER TECHNOLOGY DIFFERING FROM TRADITIONAL MEDIA?

Might these newer technologies have differing effects to those of traditional media? Malamuth and colleagues[14] have provided a theoretical viewpoint, which in the author's opinion puts the role of these newer technologies in perspective relative to more traditional media such as television. It also begins to give some insight into why cyberbullying has become more of a potential risk and a focus of attention. According to these investigators, the Internet provides motivational, disinhibitory, and opportunity aspects that make it somewhat different to traditional media in terms of its potential risk impact.

In terms of motivation the Internet is ubiquitous, in that it is always on and can easily be accessed, thus leading to high levels of exposure. There is little parental supervision, and media use today is essentially round-the-clock. The increase of media in the bedroom and the portability of new technologies (eg, smartphones) makes access almost universal. In the world of new technology there is no "family-viewing hour." Because online activities are often more interactive and engaging, users have the ability to increase their learning of both positive and negative attitudes and behaviors.

The disinhibitory aspect implies that the content is often unregulated, which is true given its global reach. Governmental constraints or filters are often short lived, given ever-expanding technological advances to get around these constraints. Studies suggest that extreme forms of violent or sexual content are more prevalent on the Internet than in other popular media.[4,15] Given that participation is private and anonymous, it allows for the searching of materials a child or adolescent would normally not do with traditional media. Anonymity has a strong influence on reducing inhibitions. Finally, online media exposure is much more difficult for parents to monitor than is media exposure in traditional venues.

Opportunity aspects play a more important role in the area of cyberbullying and child sexual exploitation. Potential victims are readily available, and the identity of the aggressor is often unknown. Often aggressors can disguise themselves, as is the case with pedophiles.

THE INTERNET AS A MEDIUM FOR VIOLENCE

Given these changes in technology, how does having access to the Internet affect a child's or adolescents exposure to violence, and in particular for this article, cyberbullying? **Fig. 3** shows how this might be conceptualized, in terms of both the Internet generally and the use of new technologies such as mobile phones, and the place of cyberbullying in this conceptualization.

The Internet, and all the platforms and devices through which it can be accessed, allows the individual to view traditional television/film and video games through live streaming or downloads. For the child or adolescent, access to what might be considered restricted materials (adult rated) is much easier via both legal and "illegal" outlets. The article by Strasburger and colleagues in this issue examines the effects of media violence in both traditional television/film and video games. It is beyond question that newer technologies have not only expanded the realm of materials but also the sources for viewing.[6]

As already noted, the motivation and disinhibitions once relegated to traditional media have been substantially changed. As the Kaiser survey found, television content is now part of a multitude of mobile devices and is more readily available.[8] There are several theoretical reasons to expect even stronger effects from exposure to violence with new technologies. The ability for interaction, rehearsal, repetitiveness, privacy, and other mechanisms all suggest that effects would be enhanced.[12]

The Internet and its varying Web sites offer another dimension. Web sites offer not only the prospect of viewing more severe violence (eg, real decapitations and executions) but also access to hate and terrorist groups. Some online archives provide instructions for making bombs or other weapons. In an extensive survey of European

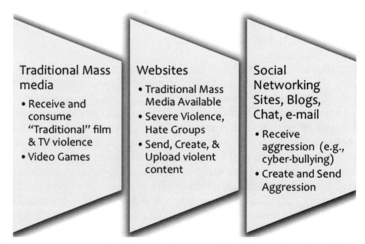

Fig. 3. The Internet, new technology, and mass media violence. (*Reprinted from* Donnerstein E. The media and aggression: from TV to the Internet. In: Forgas J, Kruglanski A, Williams K, editors. The psychology of social conflict and aggression. New York: Psychology Press; 2011. p. 275. Copyright © Psychology Press; with permission.)

countries, the EU Kids Online 2011 project[16] found that seeing graphic violent or hateful content was experienced by approximately one-third of teenagers, making it one of the higher risk concerns.

Not only can adolescents view violence on the Internet but they can also create and upload violent materials. The viewer is no longer a passive participant but now becomes the creator of violent images. Users furthermore have the ability to place that material across the globe instantaneously. Finally, Web sites, and in particular social networking sites, blogs, chat rooms, and e-mail, allow not only for the creation of aggression, but also the ability to actually aggress against another, in what has been termed cyberbullying. This aspect of the Internet and new technology is new and of increasing concern.

CYBERBULLYING

One of the issues over the years that has become of paramount concern is the use of the Internet in terms of aggressing or harassing others. This behavior is referred to as cyberbullying, which is an umbrella term related to constructs such as online bullying, electronic aggression, and Internet harassment. Cyberbullying can be defined as "any behavior performed through electronic or digital media by individuals or groups that repeatedly communicates hostile or aggressive messages intended to inflict harm or discomfort on others."[17] In their Policy Statement on violence prevention, the American Academy of Pediatrics referred to Cyberbullying as follows:

> The emergence of portable technologies, such as cellular telephones, digital cameras, and personal digital assistants and ready accessibility to social networking Internet sites has led to the advent of technology-assisted bullying behavior—a phenomenon known as "cyberbullying."[18]

There have been numerous discussions of the types of behaviors that constitute Cyberbullying. The following list involves behaviors that most agree are relevant:

1. Sending unsolicited and/or threatening e-mail
2. Spreading rumors about someone
3. Making inflammatory comments about another person in public discussion areas
4. Impersonating the victim online by sending messages that cause others to respond negatively to this individual
5. Harassing the victim during a live chat or leaving abusive messages on Web pages about the victim
6. Encouraging others to send the victim unsolicited and/or threatening e-mail
7. Leaving abusive messages on Web site guest books
8. Sending the victim pornography or other knowingly offensive graphic material.

Surveys in the United States, Europe, and Australia have indicated that somewhere between 10% and 35% of teens report being bullied online.[12] More interesting is the finding that between 10% and 20% actually admit to bullying others. In terms of gender differences there are very few, as girls are just as likely as males to be involved in cyberbullying behavior.[4] In fact, in their 10-year study of youth victimization, Jones and colleagues[19] found that while sexual solicitations and unwanted exposure to pornography had decreased, the perpetration of online harassment had increased over the 10-year period, with girls accounting for much of this increase. Also of interest in this study is the increased use of victimization via text messaging (**Fig. 4**). One should note that school is still by far the most common place where youth report being bullied.[12] While Internet bullying rates remain lower than traditional bullying, in the most recent study from the European Union,[16] being bullied online is the Internet

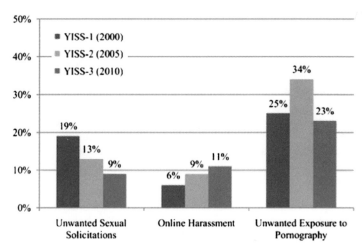

Fig. 4. Trends in unwanted experiences on the Internet for youth: YISS-1 (2000), YISS-2 (2005), and YISS-3 (2010). (*Reprinted from* Jones LM, Mitchell KJ, Finkelhor D. Trends in youth Internet victimization: findings from three youth Internet safety surveys 2000–2010. J Adolesc Health 2011;50:182. Copyright © Elsevier; with permission.)

risk that upsets youth the most. Online victims also reported elevated rates of trauma symptomatology, delinquency, and life adversity.[20]

Research on the occurrence of cyberbullying has also revealed some other interesting findings:

1. 26% have been harassed through their cell phone by voice calls or text messages[7]
2. Social network users are also more likely to report online harassment[21]
3. 34% of teens indicate that they are distressed by online harassment, and those teens who are "heavy" Internet users report more distress[22]

One of the interesting aspects of this type of harassment is the use of slurs and derogatory remarks against another. The use of gay slurs, the "N" word, or other derogatory comments seems to be all too common. Even so, one recent youth survey found that these types of remarks are often not seen as harmful by perpetrators. In this study[23] it was fond that:

1. 71% report people are more likely to use slurs online or in text messages than in person, and only about half say they are likely to ask someone using such language online to stop
2. 51% of those surveyed say they see people being mean to others on social networking sites such as Facebook and MySpace
3. 57% say "trying to be funny" is a big reason people use discriminatory language online.

Not unexpectedly, those who are the recipients of these slurs find them hurtful and harassing.

One question to be asked is why use online technology to bully someone, rather than some form of face-to-face encounter? Tokunaga[17] has offered several suggestions as to why individuals might engage in cyberbullying rather than with traditional forms of bullying, and these fit with the theoretical mechanisms of motivation, disinhibition, and opportunity discussed earlier.

First, there is anonymity offered through electronic media. The importance of anonymity in reducing inhibitions plays a significant role in many forms of aggression, and certainly cyberbullying is no exception. The process of not directly seeing one's victim and not readily being identified can intensify the motivations to harass. Second, it is an opportunistic offense, because the resulting harm can occur without any actual physical interaction. It can take place at any time of day or night from any location. Third, there is for the most part a lack of supervision or observance by others, and the act can require little if any planning. Being an anonymous, disguised perpetrator makes the threat of being caught less likely. Finally, there is accessibility; victims can be reached through several electronic devices such as cellular phones, e-mail, and instant messaging, around the clock and around the globe. As noted earlier, the Internet is ubiquitous.

EFFECTS OF CYBERBULLYING

The effects of being a victim of cyberbullying are often the same for youth who are bullied in person, which includes such consequences as a drop in grades, lower self-esteem, or depression.[24] Internet bullying shares common predictors with verbal and, to some extent, physical bullying. Recent research suggests that the effects of depression deriving from cyberbullying in adolescents might even be stronger **(Fig. 5)**.[25] This research reveals that:

1. Youth who were frequently involved with bullying behaviors, regardless of the type of bullying involved, reported higher depression scores than did youth only occasionally involved with such behaviors.
2. Cyber victims reported higher depression than bullies or bully-victims, which was not found in any other form of bullying.
3. Cyber victims may be more likely to feel isolated, dehumanized, or helpless at the time of the attack.

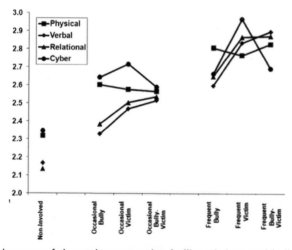

Fig. 5. Adjusted means of depression comparing bullies, victims, and bully-victims within occasionally involved and frequently involved groups. (*Reprinted from* Wang J, Nansel T, Iannotti R. Cyber and traditional bullying: differential association with depression. J Adolesc Health 2010;48:416. Copyright © Elsevier; with permission.)

These results are recent and interesting. While they strongly suggest that being an online victim has many of the same negative outcomes as traditional bullying, there is also the implication that the effects might be even more severe. There are several potential reasons why the influence of cyberbullying might be harsher on its victims.[17]

First, the place the child considers to be the most secure, the home and even the bedroom, has now become a place where he or she can be a victim. Perhaps equally important, the potential for victimization is present at all times day and night. Second, because of the anonymity of the aggressor and the inability to see the victim's reactions, effects can be perceived as harsher and more threatening. Third, effects can be "forever" in cyberspace. Postings on blogs, Web sites, or chat rooms are difficult to remove, and they maintain and prolong the consequences. Finally, for some individuals it may seem totally inescapable because being online for many children and adolescents is where these individuals socialize and interact with friends. Therefore, it often becomes very difficult to escape from potential online bullying.

An important question that parents, counselors, and practitioners might ask is: are there any warning signs that someone might be experiencing cyberbullying? Recent discussions about this issue have been considered by groups such as Education. com.[26] Many of these warning signs are similar to more traditional bullying, such as:

- Displaying numerous negative feelings, including sadness, anger, frustration, reduced tolerance, and worry
- School grades beginning to decline
- Lack of eating or sleeping
- Withdrawing from family and friends, or being reluctant to attend school and social events.

However, there are some unique characteristics that are associated with the technology involved. For example:

- Avoiding the computer, cell phone, and other technological devices
- Appearing stressed when receiving an e-mail, instant message, or text
- Avoiding conversations about computer use.

All of these behaviors tend to suggest that being harassed online might be of concern.

SUMMARY AND SOLUTIONS

Cyberbullying is somewhat recent, and is a concern that only a few years ago would have been almost entirely absent from discussion. However, technology has changed and is evolving more rapidly. The use of smartphones and social networking sites are a recent phenomenon of only the last 5 years or so. There are several more recent issues regarding new technology and children that have become of concern. These newer technologies and their emergence in the lives of children and adolescents have begun to lead us to examine areas of risk that years ago were never in our vocabulary. Besides cyberbullying, sexting, driving while texting, Facebook depression, and Internet addiction are but a few aspects emerging as areas of research and discussion.

In thinking about potential solutions to these issues, governmental regulation is an unlikely answer, particularly on a media platform that is global in nature. Rating systems might help somewhat if handled adequately, but such systems are rarely used by parents and have not been effective even with simple technology such as television and the V-chip. However, some suggestions have been made as to how this system might be more effective.[27]

As discussed in the opening article of this issue by Strasburger and colleagues, parental involvement, media literacy, and other educational initiatives seem the most likely to succeed. With respect to online risks such as cyberbullying, recent suggestions by the American Academy of Pediatrics[5] seem both reasonable and important to consider. These suggestions include:

1. Parents need to open up discussions with their younger children and adolescents about their online use and the specific issues face by today's online kids.
2. Parents need to become better educated about the many technologies their youngsters are using, and to fully understand both the positive and negatives sides of the Internet
3. Families should have an online-use plan that involves discussions of online topics and checks of privacy settings.
4. Parents should supervise online activities through active participation and communication, as opposed to remote monitoring with a "net-nanny" program (software used to monitor the Internet in the absence of parents).

There have also been suggestions that intervention and prevention programs need to go beyond merely a focus on the Internet exclusively. As Mitchell and colleagues[28] note, "Internet safety educators need to appreciate that many online victims may be at risk not because they are naive about the Internet, but because they face complicated problems resulting from more pervasive experiences of victimization and adversity." These investigators are quite correct, and intervention programs and education on media literacy need to consider the totality of the child's and adolescent's environment.

In a recent editorial in the *Journal of Adolescent Health*, Hertz and David-Ferdon[29] offer good insight into how we might focus on the issue of cyberbullying in terms of education and prevention:

> *Although bullying prevention strategies abound, there is mixed evidence of their effectiveness in changing bullying behavior among youth in the United States. However, there is evidence that comprehensive youth violence prevention programs can decrease aggressive behavior and increase prosocial behaviors. Therefore, despite the temptation to address new manifestations of youth aggression, such as online victimization, with new programs, we echo the call by Mitchell et al. to consider the context in which online victimization occurs, and suggest that researchers examine online related outcomes for existing evidence-based violence prevention programs. Given the interaction between online and in-person victimization and perpetration, researchers and practitioners should examine the effectiveness of existing evidence-based youth violence prevention programs in preventing online and in-person aggression.[29]*

The era of new technology and its influence on health-related issues for children and adolescents are firmly confronting us and changing almost daily. Many of the articles in this issue speak to the ever rapidly evolving media environment for today's youth. (See article by Strasburger and colleagues elsewhere in this issue for further exploration of this topic.) Fortunately, excellent methodologies and theoretical perspectives are available to not only understand these changes but also educate parents, practitioners, and ourselves.

When thinking about these newer technologies, one should keep in mind what Huesmann notes about the decades of research and theory on traditional media.[30] This extensive research and development of theory has provided significant insights into the role new technology will play in the development and mitigation of aggressive behavior such as cyberbullying. As Huesmann and others have noted, "the technology conduit may be changing, but the influential processes (eg, priming, activation and desensitization) may be the same."[24]

REFERENCES

1. Strasburger VC, Council on Communications and Media. Media violence (policy statement). Pediatrics 2009;124:1495–503.
2. Strasburger VC, Council on Communications and Media. Children, adolescents, and advertising (policy statement). Pediatrics 2006;118:2563–9.
3. Strasburger VC, Council on Communications and Media. Sexuality, contraception, and the media (policy statement). Pediatrics 2010;126:576–82.
4. Donnerstein E. The media and aggression: from TV to the internet. In: Forgas J, Kruglanski A, Williams K, editors. The psychology of social conflict and aggression. New York: Psychology Press; 2011. p. 267–84.
5. O'Keefe GS, Clarke-Pearson K, Council on Communications and Media. Clinical report: the impact of social media on children, adolescents, and families. Pediatrics 2011;127:800–4.
6. Gutnick AL, Robb M, Takeuchi L, et al. Always connected: the new digital media habits of young children. New York: The Joan Ganz Cooney Center at Sesame Street Workshop; 2010.
7. Lenhart A, Ling R, Campbell S, et al. Teens and mobile phones. Washington, DC: Pew Internet & American Life Project; 2010.
8. Rideout V. Generation M2: media in the lives of 8- to 18-year-olds. Menlo Park (CA): Kaiser Family Foundation; 2010.
9. Arbitron. The infinite dial 2011: Navigating digital platforms. Available at: http://www.arbitron.com/study/digital_radio_study.asp. Accessed February 2, 2012.
10. Livingstone S, Haddon L. EU kids online: final report. London: LSE; 2009. EU Kids Online.
11. Donnerstein E. The internet. In: Strasburger VC, Wilson BJ, Jordan AB. Children, adolescents, and the media. 3rd edition. Thousand Oaks (CA): Sage, in press.
12. Donnerstein E. The Internet as "fast and furious" content. In: Warburton W, Braunstein D, editors. Growing up fast and furious. Sydney (New South Wales): The Federation Press, in press.
13. Strasburger VC, Jordan AB, Donnerstein E. Health effects of media on children and adolescents. Pediatrics 2010;125:756–67.
14. Malamuth N, Linz D, Yao MZ. The Internet and aggression: motivation, disinhibitory and opportunity aspects. In: Amichai-Hamburger Y, editor. The social net: human behavior in cyberspace. New York: Oxford University Press; 2005. p. 163–91.
15. Wright PJ, Malamuth NM, Donnerstein E. Research on sex in the media: what do we know about effects on children and adolescents? In: Singer DG, Singer JL, editors. Handbook of children and the media. 2nd edition. Los Angeles (CA): Sage; 2012. p. 273–302.
16. Livingstone S, Haddon L, Görzig A, et al. Risks and safety on the internet: the perspective of European children. Full findings. London: LSE; 2011. EU Kids Online.
17. Tokunaga R. Following you home from school: a critical review and synthesis of research on cyberbullying victimization. Comput Hum Behav 2010;26:277–87.
18. American Academy of Pediatrics Committee on Injury, Violence, and Poison Prevention. Role of the pediatrician in youth violence. Pediatrics 2009;124:393–402.
19. Jones LM, Mitchell KJ, Finkelhor D. Trends in youth internet victimization: findings from three youth internet safety surveys 2000-2010. J Adolesc Health 2011;50:179–86.

20. Mitchell KJ, Jones LM, Finkelhor D, et al. Youth internet safety survey. Durham (NH): Crimes against Children Research Center, University of New Hampshire; 2011.

21. Lenhart A. Cyberbullying: what the research is telling us. Washington, DC: Pew Internet & American Life Project; 2009.

22. Wolak J, Mitchell KJ, Finkelhor D. Unwanted and wanted exposure to online pornography in a national sample of youth internet. Pediatrics 2007;119:247–57.

23. Associated Press-MTV digital abuse survey. 2011. Available at: http://surveys.ap.org/data/KnowledgeNetworks/AP_DigitalAbuseSurvey_ToplineTREND_1st%20story.pdf. Accessed February 2, 2012.

24. Ferdon CD, Hertz MF. Electronic media, violence, and adolescents: an emerging public health problem. J Adolesc Health 2007;41:S1–5.

25. Wang J, Nansel T, Iannotti R. Cyber and traditional bullying: differential association with depression. J Adolesc Health 2010;48:415–7.

26. What are the signs that my child is being bullied online? Available at: Education.Com; http://www.education.com/reference/article/signs-child-bullied-online. Accessed February 2, 2012.

27. Gentile DA. The rating systems for media products. In: Calvert S, Wilson B, editors. Handbook on children and media. Boston: Blackwell; 2007. p. 527–51.

28. Mitchell KJ, Finkelhor D, Wolak J, et al. Youth internet victimization in a broader victimization context. J Adolesc Health 2011;48:128–34.

29. Hertz MF, David-Ferdon C. Online aggression: a reflection of in-person victimization or a unique phenomenon? J Adolesc Health 2011;48:119–20.

30. Huesmann RL. The impact of electronic media violence: scientific theory and research. J Adolesc Health 2007;41:S6–13.

Prosocial Effects of Media

Marjorie J. Hogan, MD

KEYWORDS

- Prosocial media • Prosocial behavior • Coviewing • Content analysis
- General learning model • Media education

KEY POINTS

- Caring adults worry about the harmful influences of media exposure and how to recognize and encourage positive and healthy use of media.
- Media are not intrinsically good or bad; content, context, and coviewing are all important variables.
- Parents and other adults can optimize the messages from positive programs by encouraging discussion and even role playing about the lessons in the programs.
- Adolescents are prime targets for health messages via various media platforms.

Children and teens grow up in a world permeated by media: in their homes, at school, with friends, or solo during leisure hours. Parents, teachers, health care providers, and other caring adults worry about the harmful influence of media messages and images on young minds and also wonder how to recognize and encourage positive and healthy use of media.

For decades, experts have commented on the power of media. For example, in 1973, Federal Communication Commission chairperson Johnson stated: "…all television is educational television. The only question is, what is it teaching?"[1] Based on a rich body of research, we know that media depictions can lead to negative attitudes and behavior in some young viewers. Could prosocial, tolerant, and cooperative attitudes and behavior also be learned and imitated by children and adolescents? Can media nurture or stimulate creativity or actively promote health and well-being in young consumers?

PROSOCIAL MEDIA

Research on prosocial media suffers from the lack of a definition, not only of what constitutes prosocial content in media but also how to measure prosocial outcomes. For the Children's Television Act of 1990, legislators arrived at the definition of

Department of Pediatrics, Hennepin County Medical Center, 701 Park Avenue, Green 7, Minneapolis, MN 55415, USA
E-mail address: hogan003@umn.edu

Pediatr Clin N Am 59 (2012) 635–645
doi:10.1016/j.pcl.2012.03.020
0031-3955/12/$ – see front matter © 2012 Elsevier Inc. All rights reserved.

programming that "further(s) the positive development of the child in any respect, including the child's cognitive/intellectual or emotional/social needs."[2]

Mares and Woodward[3] define prosocial content and effects more precisely as friendly play, inclusiveness, aggression reduction, altruism, and stereotype reduction. Prosocial content has "the potential for fostering social interactions that are nonviolent and positive in tone"[4] or can "encourage or enable children to interact with each other in friendly, inclusive ways."[3] Wilson[5] defines prosocial behavior as voluntary behavior intended to benefit someone else. Gentile and Crick (Douglas Gentile, University of Iowa, personal communication, May 2006) devised a prosocial scale using peer nomination:

- Who does nice things for others?
- Who tried to cheer up other kids who are upset or sad about something and makes them feel happy again?

CONTENT ANALYSIS

"Media are not intrinsically good or bad."[6] Content, context, and coviewing are all important variables. Few programs are created with prosocial modeling for child viewers in mind; however, we know that children often view adult-themed programming, situation comedies, reality television, and other adult fare. Content analyses confirm that most prosocial shows (72% for children) are on public television and are aimed at children less than 5 years of age.[4] "Therefore, the most important question is not how much prosocial content there is in children's programming, but how much there is in adult programming that children are likely to watch."[4–6]

Content analyses several years ago found that few mainstream television programs featured prosocial content: 4 of 20 programs in 1999 had prosocial messages and only 2 of the most popular programs in 2001 portrayed friendliness, altruism, or aggression reduction.[4] Children's programming during this time did better, with 50% of children's shows containing at least 1 prosocial lesson.[7] Smith and colleagues in 2006[8] sampled content from 2227 programs over many channels and found that 73% of the programs had 2.92 helping or sharing incidents per hour. Most incidents involved White males and many had a humorous, realistic, or rewarded context. Dedicated children's programming had just more than 4 altruistic incidents per hour. Comparing broadcast television with the National Television Violence Study, children were more likely to see altruism (3 of 4 shows) than violence (2 of 3 shows), but they view altruistic events only 3 times per hour compared with 6 violent events per hour. In children's programming, violent events occur more than 3 times more often than altruistic events, so an average American child watching 3 hours of children's programming daily see 4380 acts of altruism and 15,330 act of violence annually.[5]

HOW CHILDREN AND TEENS USE MEDIA

Children and teens spend a lot of time with media, significantly more in the Kaiser Foundation's 2010 survey compared with the 2006 data.[9] On average, 7 hours 38 minutes daily are devoted to media use: 53 hours weekly for 8-year-olds to 18-year-olds. Because these youth are skillful multitaskers, "they pack a total of 10 hours and 45 minutes into those 7 1/2 hours."[9] Since the last survey, use of every form of media (television, video games, computers, and music) has increased, with the exception of reading. This increase in media use is fueled by an explosion in online and mobile media, notably cell phones, iPods, handheld video players, laptops, and now, iPads and other similar multiuse platforms. In the Kaiser survey, 71% of children and teens have a television in their bedroom; many of these have cable or satellite access. Most 8-year-olds to 18-year-olds report no parental rules about media content or time limits, with the exception of computer use. Whether anyone is watching or not, 64% of homes have the television on during meals and 45% leave the set on virtually all of the time.[9] "For many families, media use has become part of the fabric of daily life."[10]

RESEARCH ON PROSOCIAL MEDIA AND IMPACT ON CHILDREN

Negative effects related to media messages and images are the result of 2 mechanisms:

- Children learn how to do things (and whether behavior is appropriate) by observation, incorporating scripts into their behavioral repertoire
- Emotional responses to media images and messages affect responses to real-life events.

Intuitively, these mechanisms could also encourage prosocial attitudes and behavior. The General Learning Model[11,12] describes "various pathways by which both prosocial and antisocial learning from the media can occur."[3] Children and teens may imitate positive behaviors, draw on scripts for use in similar situations, and show certain emotional responses to compelling, positive media images.

The bulk of research on prosocial media is 20 to 30 years old and there are no longitudinal studies in the literature. In addition, this research involves only television (although television is still the most used of the mass media for all age groups):

If observational learning from TV has such striking and lasting antisocial consequences, it is reasonable to expect that the medium also has the potential for modifying behavior in desirable, prosocial directions. Recent studies in laboratory and naturalistic settings have provided evidence supportive of this hypothesis, although the correlations are not generally as strong or as clear as those between viewing TV violence and subsequent aggressive behavior.[13]

Mares and Woodward[3,4] reviewed research on programming not intended for young audiences in terms of prosocial content, but limitations included definitional ambiguity of prosocial, both of programming and outcomes (most studies measured educational or cognitive rather than social outcomes). A variety of field or naturalistic studies observed young children's behaviors after exposure to televised prosocial content, compared with children watching programs with aggressive or neutral themes, and generally found trends toward more cooperative interaction or helping behavior. The longevity and robustness of the behaviors could not be analyzed given the design of the studies.[14–17]

Correlational studies (analyzing which programs children self-select at home) do not help in the understanding of causality: do prosocial programs influence children to behave in a more cooperative, positive manner or do prosocial children choose programs with positive content? Are there other variables, including gender, parent influence, or socioeconomic status? Older research again suggested a relationship between educational or prosocial content and positive behaviors.[18,19]

More robust studies, although few, include meta-analyses and longitudinal designs.

- A meta-analysis of 230 studies carried out before 1978[20] showed prosocial effects (book buying, library card use, safety, and conservation activism) to be twice as strong as antisocial effects (aggression, criminality, stereotyping) of media viewing. Both in laboratory and in naturalistic settings, the prosocial effects were more enduring.

- Another meta-analysis, in 1994,[21] found antisocial and prosocial effects of media viewing to be equivalent.
- The most recent meta-analysis[22] evaluated 34 studies after 1978 for positive interaction, aggression reduction, altruism, and stereotype reduction. Prosocial media have a weak to moderate effect, strongest for altruism. As a result, the "best guess is that the effects of violent content and prosocial content are reasonably close in magnitude, though violent content may be somewhat more powerful."
- An impressive longitudinal study from the University of Iowa[23] measured the long-term association between violence and educational media exposure, both in terms of the subtypes of aggressive behavior and prosocial behavior. Study results suggest that both violent and educational media affect young children and lead to mainly relational aggression for young girls and physical aggression for boys. "Identification with same-gender television and media characters is a key component of this process." Parental monitoring of media use was negatively associated with aggression for both girls and boys. In this study, educational programming was not associated with positive behaviors, and the association with relational aggression suggests that not only is content important but also that excessive media consumption (of any genre) can have negative consequences for peer interaction. Relational aggression may be modeled in an educational program and misconstrued. For example, children may be shown excluding others in the playground only to reconcile at the end of the program; the investigators note that some young children may miss this lesson, having age-appropriate difficulty understanding plots.[23]

These studies suggest that "for young children, viewing prosocial TV per se facilitates acquisition or enhancement of prosocial behavior"; however, "the influences are not as powerful or direct as influences of specially-designed school programs, training in role playing, or a combination of prosocial TV, role-playing and verbal labeling."[13] Perhaps prosocial actions modeled on television are "less salient for young children or less attention-grabbing than active participation in role playing and discussion. Young children are less likely to think about or remember the messages of the programs or make inferences or generalizations."[13] The "results of experimental interventions in which viewing is accompanied by related activities and curriculum are generally encouraging, particularly in comparison to the weaker or nonexistent effects observed without additional materials."[3] So, parents and other adults can optimize the messages from positive television programs by encouraging discussion and even role playing about the lessons of the programming.

RESEARCH ON CHILDREN'S PROGRAMMING

Many Public Broadcasting Service productions, as well as some designed by Disney and Nickelodeon, "meet the social and emotional needs of children"[4] and experts opine that prosocial values and behavior can be modeled and taught through thoughtful programming.[24,25] These programs include the well-known Sesame Street, Mister Rogers' Neighborhood, Electric Company, Arthur, and Barney and Friends.

Sesame Street, initially developed to enhance preschoolers' cognitive ability, incorporated additional goals to encourage prosocial attitudes and behavior, specifically tolerance, cooperation, and friendliness. Fisch and Truglio[26] acknowledge that television has documented effects on children's behavior, both prosocial and antisocial, but for unclear reasons found that children were less able to generalize modeled prosocial behavior to new situations than they were able to imitate behavior in a context and situation like that modeled on the screen. One-time exposure to a prosocial scene was not sufficient for behavioral change; apparently, repeated exposure to prosocial behavior is necessary for positive effects to occur.

- Several studies of "Sesame Street" viewership led to some predictable conclusions, although the results were not uniform. Young viewers tended to play more cooperatively, show more tolerance for others, or choose nonaggressive approaches to problem solving; some studies showed persistence of positive behaviors over time.[26–28]
- Another seminal program designed for preschoolers, "Mister Rogers' Neighborhood," focused on positive affective, social messages rather than cognitive gain. Children experienced "such positive behaviors as nurturance and sympathy, task persistence, empathy, and imaginativeness from viewing the program"[14,15,25]
- Calvert and Kotler[29] used both experimental and naturalistic methodologies to examine several prosocial programs on cable, broadcast, and public television. Elementary school-aged children learned more from these prosocial programs than from traditional school-related educational offerings, specifically being able to identify emotions of televised characters and apply lessons learned to their own experiences.[6]
- To sum up the research, Mares and Woodard[22] conducted a meta-analysis in 2005 of 34 studies on prosocial television. Their analysis involved more than 5000 children and found a medium-sized effect of .27, consistent with prosocial programming enhancing the prosocial behavior of children. The strongest effect was on altruism, with positive interaction and tolerance slightly weaker. These outcomes most likely reflect that television can more easily show helping others; cooperation or tolerance may be more abstract.[5,22]

INTERACTIVE ELECTRONIC MEDIA

Video games are increasingly popular with children and youth and constitute a multibillion dollar market.[30] According to the Kaiser Family Foundation study from 2010, 87% of youth aged 8 to 18 years old have a dedicated video game system at home and the average home has 2.3 consoles. On a typical day, 60% of these youngsters play video games and many use their cell phones or handheld video game devices.[9] A growing body of behavioral science research has shown a link between playing violent video games and aggressive attitudes and behavior, similar to that between television viewing and aggression-related outcomes.[31] In parallel with knowledge about prosocial television programming, research is emerging about a relationship between playing video games modeling prosocial situations and behaviors. A relevant series of 3 studies by Gentile and colleagues[32] at the University of Iowa found the amount of prosocial game play to be "positively related to helping behavior, cooperation and sharing, and empathy."

- The experimental study randomized children to play a prosocial, aggressive, or neutral video game; those playing the prosocial game were significantly more likely to help a child win a gift certificate.
- The longitudinal study looked at prosocial behaviors in a large cohort of Japanese students playing video games after 3 to 4 months and found that exposure to prosocial games at time 1 led to increased positive behaviors at time 2.

- A cross-sectional design studied the video game habits and prosocial attributes of Singaporean high-school students. After controlling for several variables, the students playing prosocial video games had more helping behavior, cooperation and sharing, and empathy. Violent video game play was positively related to hostile attribution bias and negatively related to helping behavior.

Studies have shown that playing violent video games does lead to decreased prosocial behavior.

- In a study of 100 elementary schoolchildren,[33] exposure to video game violence was related to lower measures of empathy when compared with both real-life violence and other forms of entertainment violence. For the investigators, this finding of decreased empathy raised concerns about desensitization to violence: an outcome possibly unique to this medium "because of the active nature of playing video games, intense engagement, and the tendency to be translated into fantasy play."
- A meta-analysis of 35 studies from the University of Iowa[31] found increased aggression and decreased prosocial behavior in children and young adults after exposure to video game violence, concluding that "exposure to violent video games is negatively correlated with helping in the real world."
- A total of 224 participants played either a violent or nonviolent video game and were asked subsequently to complete a story about interpersonal conflict. Those viewing the violent video game described the protagonist as more angry and aggressive in thought and behavior.[34]
- In a follow-up study,[35] participants played a violent, prosocial, or neutral video game to examine both aggressive and prosocial effects and then completed 3 stories. The group playing violent video games wrote more aggressive endings to the stories, whereas the prosocial group produced helpful, empathetic, or supportive endings. Both this study and the previous study concluded that "playing video games creates social biases that influence feelings, attitudes, and behavior."

As Gentile and colleagues[32] conclude, "the tiny research literature on prosocial game effects mirrors the huge literature on violent game effects, supporting the idea that the same basic social-cognitive processes underlie both phenomena."

LESSONS LEARNED FROM THE RESEARCH ON PROSOCIAL MEDIA

Exposure to prosocial messages in media seems to have a greater effect on younger children; the effect peaks at about age 7 years and declines thereafter, up to age 12 years.[3,4] Most prosocial programming is aimed at the younger viewers (age 3–7 years) and this age group may well view programs with less skepticism and decreased ability to critically analyze content.[21] However, many years ago, Eisenberg and Mussen[13] mused that for older children, the impact of prosocial programming may be less overt and

> exposure to prosocial media may help foster prosocial development, at least in certain areas. Perhaps being in a more advanced stage of cognitive development, older children may pay more attention and formulate generalizations from observational learning. These generalizations may be stored in memory and subsequently serve as mediators between the child's perception of other people's needs and the child's response (help, sharing, cooperation) to those needs.

Socioeconomic status mediates response to prosocial-mediated messages; these messages seem to resonate with children from families with more educated and prosperous parents.[4]

Several studies described earlier show the importance of combining viewing of prosocial media with related lessons and activities, including role playing and age-appropriate discussion and deconstruction of messages. These activities can take place in the home or in a school setting. For some time, research has emphasized the positive role of adult coviewing (a basic tenet of media education) with "successful mediation as simple as labeling or commenting on prosocial acts."[3,4]

Questions and conundrums about prosocial media include the following:

1. Some programs combine prosocial and antisocial behavior, creating confusion in young viewers' minds; the message may be lost in the mayhem followed by a brief punishment.
2. In media violence research, behavior that is rewarded, justified, presented with humor, and involves relatable characters is more likely to be imitated. Should prosocial behavior in the media be rewarded? Should the reward be extrinsic or intrinsic? Should altruism/kindness be rewarded?
3. Is imitation of prosocial behavior short-lived? Is timing critical? What are the strategies for encouraging prosocial lessons to be incorporated over time? Would incorporation of humor, relatable characters, music, animals, or other features be more attractive for young viewers?

A FRESH LOOK AT NEW TECHNOLOGIES AND HEALTH BENEFITS

Research is emerging of the benefits of exergaming (playing video games with physical activity built into the experience). Dance, Dance Revolution, Wii Fit, and other popular exercise or dancing games bring interactivity and direct feedback to the format, supplying "operant conditioning and acting as an interactive trainer."[12] One study[36] found that these popular games potentially promote health by spurring adolescents to moderate or vigorous activity (4–8 times resting energy expenditure). Given our national epidemic of youth obesity, finding that youth with increased body mass index (calculated as weight in kilograms divided by the square of height in meters) enjoyed the exergames more than their slimmer peers is encouraging. A 2009 eating disorders prevention program used 8 media literacy sessions with more than 500 middle-school students. When compared with a control group, youth in the media literacy group showed a decrease in shape and weight concern, dieting, body dissatisfaction, ineffectiveness, and depression. This study suggests that media literacy can be an effective intervention for reducing eating disorder risk factors.[37] Knowing that excessive time spent with screen media is a risk factor for obesity, Schmidt and colleagues[38] sought strategies for reducing media time by reviewing existing studies. Twenty-nine of 47 studies achieved significant reduction in screen media time with children less than 12 years of age. Successful strategies included electronic monitoring devices, contingent feedback systems, or clinic-based counseling. More studies are needed to examine longevity of lifestyle changes and health outcomes.[39]

Adolescents eagerly use media in all its forms and are a prime target for health messages via different media platforms. Most still consider family and friends to be trusted sources for health facts, but for information on hot-button issues, including birth control, pregnancy, and sexually transmitted infections (STIs), teens often turn to Google.[40] Providing them with responsible online sites (Planned Parenthood, Go

Ask Alice) allows teens to seek crucial information and guidance privately and in real time. New technologies are full of possibilities for enhancing the health of teens, from text messaging safe-sex information to STI results.[41] Teens spend lots of time playing video games, so new computer games like The Baby Game and It's your Game: Keep it Real are potentially powerful tools in the quest to decrease teen pregnancy by increasing knowledge and changing attitudes about unsafe sex. In California, adolescents who use cell phones may receive text messages from Hook Up (a state-wide low-cost service to facilitate access to information and health care) for reproductive health and referrals to youth-oriented clinic services; as of 2009, more than 3000 youth had signed-up for Hook Up.[42] TeenSource offers Web-based information and posts videos on YouTube aimed at prevention of teen pregnancy. Evidence of long-term (and even short-term) benefits (eg, for health) from new technologies is lacking, but the potential is real and exciting. "As digital technologies rapidly evolve, great opportunity exists for health care professionals to develop and leverage these new technologies to improve learning around sexual and reproductive health and change risk-taking behaviors and attitudes of youth and young adults."[40]

Adolescents love music and spend many hours listening to tunes on iPods and other devices.[9] A 2009 article[43] reviewed 4 studies and found that listening to songs with pro-social (as opposed to neutral) lyrics increased helping behaviors. This positive effect is mediated by empathy and provides support for the general learning model.[11,12] The author argues that "increasing exposure to prosocial music and decreasing exposure to antisocial music could significantly benefit social encounters."[43]

ROLES OF PARENTS AND OTHER ADULT MONITORS OF MEDIA HABITS

As recommended by the American Academy of Pediatrics (AAP) and other advocacy groups, parents are strongly encouraged to be monitors and models of healthy media habits for their children and adolescents. Encouraging parents and other involved adults to educate and involve themselves in the media lives of young people allows prosocial programming to be identified, emphasized, and used appropriately for both education and entertainment. Parents' goal should be teaching, modeling, and reinforcing media literacy; this allows negative media images and messages to be neutralized and positive, prosocial media lessons to be identified and embraced. The basic tenets of media education or media literacy include the following[44]:

1. All media images and messages are created
2. Each form of media uses its own techniques and language
3. No 2 people experience media the same way
4. Media have economic, political, and social contexts
5. Each media message has its own values and points of view.

Parents are uniquely positioned to guide their children's media use, creating lifelong positive habits through encouraging media literacy. Parents are not only their own children's cultural teachers but know each child's strengths, interests, and vulnerabilities. "Parents understand the importance of family priorities and beliefs and how media messages and images affect the family."[42] The AAP, through its various media-related policy statements recommends the following measures to optimize media use habits within families[45,46]:

1. Limit media use to 1 to 2 quality hours daily
2. Avoid media exposure for children less than the age of 2 years
3. Make wise media choices for the family

4. Arrange your home to be a positive media environment; for example, keep media out of children's bedrooms and turn off television during family meals
5. Coview media with children and teens; critical viewing and critical thinking are cornerstones of media literacy
6. Incorporate media education into children's daily lives
7. Be a positive media role-model
8. Be an advocate and activist for healthy, positive media for children
9. Emphasize alternative activities: music, reading, active, physical play, creativity, unscripted playtime.

SUMMARY

An old quote is relevant: "inevitably, children will be influenced by what they see and hear on television, for television arouses emotions, communicates values, norms and standards, and provides models whose actions will be imitated – all factors that modify a child's behavior."[13] In our new millennium, television is only part of the equation. On the individual, family, and community level, strengthening communication skills, relationships, and tolerance and fostering empathy and altruism are vital for coping and thriving. With the conviction that media will continue to evolve in complexity and become more interwoven into our lives, what will media teach and model?[47]

REFERENCES

1. Liebert RM, Neale JM, Davidson ES. The early window: effects of television on children and youth. New York: Pergamon Press; 1973.
2. Federal Communications Commission. Policies and rules concerning children's television programming. FCC Record 1991;6:2111–27.
3. Mares ML, Woodard EH. Effects of prosocial media content on children's social interactions. In: Singer DG, Singer JL, editors. Handbook of children and the media. 2nd edition. Thousand Oaks (CA): Sage; 2012. p. 197–214.
4. Mares ML, Woodard EH. Prosocial effects on children's social interactions. In: Singer DG, Singer JL, editors. Handbook of children and the media. Thousand Oaks (CA): Sage; 2001. p. 183–205.
5. Wilson BJ. Media and children's aggression, fear, and altruism. Future Child 2008;18:87–118.
6. Prosocial effects of media. In: Strasburger VC, Wilson BJ, Jordan AB, editors. Children, adolescents and the media. 2nd edition. Thousand Oaks (CA): Sage; 2009. p. 117–44.
7. Woodard EH. The 1999 state of children's television report: programming for children over broadcast and cable television (report #28). Philadelphia: Annenberg Policy Center; 1999.
8. Smith SW, Smith SL, Pieper KM, et al. Altruism of American television: examining the amount of, and context surrounding, acts of helping and sharing. J Comm 2006;56:707–27.
9. Rideout VJ, Foehr UG, Roberts DF. Generation M2: media in the lives of 8- to 18-year olds. Menlo Park (CA): Henry J. Kaiser Family Foundation; 2010.
10. Rideout VJ, Roberts DF, Foehr UG. Generation M: media in the lives of 8- to 18-year olds. Menlo Park (CA): Henry J. Kaiser Family Foundation; 2005.
11. Buckley KE, Anderson CA. A theoretical model of the effects and consequences of playing video games. In: Vorderer P, Bryant J, editors. Playing video games–motives, responses, and consequences. Mahwah (NJ): Lawrence Erlbaum; 2006. p. 363–78.

12. Anderson CA, Gentile DA, Dill KE. Prosocial, antisocial, and other effects of recreational video games. In: Singer DG, Singer JL, editors. Handbook of children and the media. 2nd edition. Thousand Oaks (CA): Sage; 2012. p. 249–72.

13. Eisenberg N, Mussen PH. The roots of prosocial behavior in children. Cambridge (United Kingdom): Cambridge; 1989.

14. Friedrich LK, Stein AH. Aggressive and prosocial television programs and the natural behavior of children. Monogr Soc Res Child Dev 1973;38:1–64.

15. Friedrich LK, Stein AH. Prosocial television and young children: the effects of verbal labeling and role-playing on development and behavior. Child Dev 1975;46:27–38.

16. Poulos RW, Rubinstein EA, Liebert RM. Positive social learning. J Comm 1975;25: 90–7.

17. Ahammer IM, Murray JP. Kindness in the kindergarten: the relative influence of role-playing and prosocial television in facilitating altruism. Int J Behav Dev 1979;2:133–57.

18. Sprafkin JN, Rubinstein EA. Children's television viewing habits and prosocial behavior: a field correlational study. J Broadcast 1979;23:265–76.

19. Rosenkatter LI. The television situation comedy and children's prosocial behavior. J Appl Soc Psychol 1999;29:979–93.

20. Hearold S. A synthesis of 1043 effects of television on social behavior. In: Comstock G, editor. Public communication and behavior, vol. 1. New York: Academic Press; 1986. p. 65–133.

21. Paik H, Comstock G. The effects of television violence on antisocial behavior: a meta-analysis. Comm Res 1994;21:516–46.

22. Mares ML, Woodard EH. Positive effects of television on children's social interaction: a meta-analysis. Media Psychol 2005;7:301–22.

23. Ostrov JM, Gentile D, Crick N. Media exposure, aggression and prosocial behavior during early childhood: a longitudinal study. Soc Dev 2006;15:612–27.

24. Rushton JP. Effects of prosocial television and film material on the behavior of viewers. In: Berkowitz L, editor. Advances in experimental psychology, vol. 10. New York: Academic Press; 1979. p. 321–51.

25. Huston AC, Donnerstein E, Fairchild H, et al. Big world, small screen: the role of television in American society. Lincoln (NE): University of Nebraska Press; 1992.

26. Fisch SM, Truglio RT. "G" is for growing: thirty years of research on children and Sesame Street. Mahwah (NJ): Lawrence Erlbaum; 2001.

27. Paulson F. Teaching cooperation on television: an evaluation of Sesame Street social goals program. AV Commun Rev 1974;22:229–46.

28. Zielinska IE, Chambers B. Using group viewing of television to teach preschool social skills. J Educ Televis 1995;21:85–99.

29. Calvert S, Kotler J. Lessons from children's television: the impact of the Children's Television Act on children's learning. Applied Developmental Psychology 2003; 24:275–335.

30. Industry facts. Entertainment Software Association. Available at: http://www.theesa.com/facts/index.asp. Accessed November 28, 2011.

31. Anderson CA, Bushman BJ. Effects of violent video games on aggressive behavior, aggressive cognition, aggressive effect, physiological arousal, and prosocial behavior: a meta-analytic review of the scientific literature. Psychol Sci 2001;12:353–9.

32. Gentile DA, Anderson CA, Yukawa S, et al. The effects of prosocial video games on prosocial behaviors: international evidence from correlational, experimental, and longitudinal studies. Pers Soc Psychol Bull 2009;35:752–63.

33. Funk JB, Baldacci HB, Pasold T, et al. Violence exposure in real-life, video games, television, movies and the Internet; is there desensitization? J Adolesc 2004;27:23–9.

34. Bushman BJ, Anderson CA. Violent video games and hostile expectations: a test of the general aggression model. Pers Soc Psychol Bull 2002;28:1679–86.

35. Narvaez D, Matten B, MacMichael D. Kill Bandits, Collect Gold or Save the Dying: the effects of playing a prosocial video game. Notre Dame (IN): University of Notre Dame, Center for Ethical Education; 2007.

36. Bailey BW, McInnis K. Energy cost of exergaming: a comparison of the energy cost of 6 forms of exergaming. Arch Pediatr Adolesc Med 2011;165:597–602.

37. Wilksch SM, Wade TD. Reduction of shape and weight concerns in young adolescents: a 30-month controlled evaluation of a media literacy program. J Am Acad Child Adolesc Psychiatry 2009;48:652–61.

38. Schmidt ME, Haines J, O'Brien A, et al. Systematic review of effective strategies for reducing screen time in young children. Obesity (Silver Spring) 2012. DOI:10.038/oby.2011.348.

39. Sallis JF. Potential versus actual benefits of exergames. Arch Pediatr Adolesc Med 2011;165:667–9.

40. Boyar R, Levine D, Zensius N. TECHsex: youth sexuality and reproductive health in the digital age. Oakland (CA): ISIS; 2011.

41. Levine D, McCright J, Dobkin L, et al. SEXINFO: a sexual health text messaging service for San Francisco youth. Am J Public Health 2008;98:1–3.

42. Carroll JA, Kirkpatrick RL. Impact of social media on adolescent behavioral health in California. Oakland (CA): Adolescent Health Collaborative; 2011.

43. Greitemeyer T. Effects of songs with prosocial lyrics on prosocial behavior: further evidence and a mediating mechanism. Pers Soc Psychol Bull 2009;35:1500–11.

44. American Academy of Pediatrics. Media education in the practice setting. Elk Grove Village (IL): Media Matters, AAP; 1999.

45. Hogan MJ. Parents and other adults: models and monitors of healthy media habits. In: Singer DG, Singer JL, editors. Handbook of children and the media. 2nd edition. Thousand Oaks (CA): Sage; 2012.

46. Council on Communications and Media. Media education. Pediatrics 2010;126: 1012–7.

47. Hogan MJ, Strasburger VC. Media and prosocial behavior in children and adolescents. In: Nucci LP, Narvaez D, editors. Handbook of moral and character education. New York: Routledge; 2008. p. 537–53.

Video Games: Good, Bad, or Other?

Sara Prot, MA*, Katelyn A. McDonald, Craig A. Anderson, PhD,
Douglas A. Gentile, PhD

KEYWORDS

- Media effects • Video games • Aggression • Prosocial behavior

KEY POINTS

- The growing popularity of video games has instigated a debate among parents, researchers, video game producers and policymakers concerning their harmful and helpful effects.
- Video games are very effective teachers that affect players in multiple domains.
- Some of these effects can be harmful (eg, effects of violent video games on aggression).
- Other video game effects can be beneficial (eg, effects of action games on visual-spatial skills).
- Video game effects are complex and would be better understood as multiple dimensions rather than a simplistic "good-bad" dichotomy.

Video games are an extremely popular pastime among children and adolescents. Today, 90% of American children and teens play video games.[1,2] On a typical day, youth play video games for an average of 2 hours.[3] Time spent playing is even higher among some segments of the population, with 25% of young males reporting playing video games for 4 hours a day or more.[4]

The rising popularity of video games has instigated a debate among parents, researchers, video game producers, and policymakers concerning potential harmful and helpful effects of video games on children. Views expressed in this debate have often been extreme, either idealizing or vilifying video games.[5–7] The critics and the proponents tend to ignore research evidence supporting the views of the opposing camps and label video games as clearly "good" or "bad."

Are video games good or bad? Several relevant findings on the effects of video games are displayed in **Table 1**. The explosion in research on video games in the past 10 years has helped increase our understanding of how video games affect players. It is clear that video games are powerful teachers that have significant effects

Department of Psychology, Iowa State University, W112 Lagomarcino Hall, Ames, IA 50011-3180, USA
* Corresponding author.
E-mail address: sprot@iastate.edu

Pediatr Clin N Am 59 (2012) 647–658
doi:10.1016/j.pcl.2012.03.016
0031-3955/12/$ – see front matter © 2012 Elsevier Inc. All rights reserved.

Table 1
Summary of main research findings on positive and negative effects of video games on players

Positive Effects	Negative Effects
Action games improve a range of visual-spatial skills[8]	Violent games
Educational games successfully teach specific knowledge and skills[9]	Increase aggressive thoughts, feelings and behaviors[13]
Exergames can improve physical activity levels[10]	Desensitize players to violence, decrease empathy and helping[14–16]
Prosocial games	Video game play is negatively related to school performance[17]
Increase empathy and helping[11]	Video games may exacerbate attention problems[18]
May decrease aggression[12]	It seems that some players can become addicted to video games[1]

in several domains, some of which could be considered beneficial and some of which could be considered harmful.[19,20]

The aim of this article is to give an overview of research findings on positive and negative effects of video games, thus providing an empirical answer to the question, "are video games good or bad?" Several negative effects of video games are reviewed first, including effects of violent video games on aggression-related variables as well as effects on attention deficits, school performance, and gaming addiction. Next, positive effects of video games are described, including effects of action games on visual-spatial skills, and effects of educational video games, exergames, and prosocial video games. Finally, some conclusions and guidelines are offered with the goal of helping pediatricians, parents, and other caregivers protect children from negative effects while maximizing the positive effects of| video games.

FIVE DIMENSIONS OF THE EFFECTS OF VIDEO GAMES

Gentile and colleagues[21–23] have proposed that video games can affect players on at least 5 dimensions (**Box 1**).

Games are multidimensional and have complex effects on players. Each dimension is likely to be associated with different effects. The amount of game play has been linked to poorer academic performance and increased risk of obesity.[24,25] Violent game content is a significant risk factor for aggression, whereas prosocial game content can increase empathy and helping, and educational games can improve specific skills.[9,11,13] The context in which games are played may alter or create new effects. For example, playing in virtual teams can encourage collaboration.[26]

Box 1
Five dimensions of the effects of video games

1. Amount of game play

2. Content of play

3. Context of the game

4. Structure of the game

5. Mechanics of game play

Research on effects of game structure shows that fast-paced action games can increase visual/spatial skills (sometimes misinterpreted as "improved attention").[27-29] Innovative game mechanics such as the interactive *Wii* controller have been successfully used to promote physical activity and have even been used for physical therapy.[10,30]

A great strength of this approach is that it offers a different way of thinking about the effects of video games that surpasses a simplistic good-versus-bad dichotomy. Video games are complex and may influence players in different ways through different learning mechanisms. Even a single video game, such as *Grand Theft Auto*, might simultaneously have positive effects on players (improved visual processing) and negative effects (increased aggressive thoughts and feelings).

NEGATIVE EFFECTS OF VIDEO GAMES
Violent Video Game Effects

By far the largest and best understood research domain concerns the effects of violent video games on aggression. Findings of experimental, correlational, and longitudinal studies confirm that video game violence can significantly increase aggressive thoughts, emotions, and behavior over both the short term and the long term.[13,17]

Although there are differing opinions about the strength of the data, a recent comprehensive meta-analytical review examined effects of violent video games on 6 relevant outcomes (aggressive behavior, aggressive cognition, aggressive affect, physiological arousal, empathy, and prosocial behavior).[13] The meta-analysis included 136 research articles with 381 effect-size estimates involving more than 130,000 participants. This large sample included both published and unpublished studies from Eastern and Western cultures. The main findings of the meta-analysis are shown in **Fig. 1**. Video game play had significant effects on all 6 outcomes. Exposure to violent video games can be seen as a causal risk factor for increased aggressive behavior, cognition, and affect, with reduced empathy and prosocial behavior.

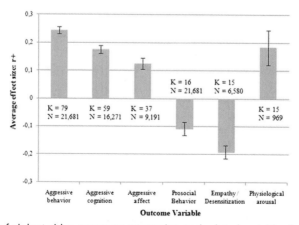

Fig. 1. Effects of violent video games on aggression and related variables (results from the "Best raw" sample). K, number of effects; N, total sample size. Vertical capped bars are the upper and lower 95% confidence intervals. (*From* Anderson CA, Shibuya A, Ihori N, et al. Violent video game effects on aggression, empathy, and prosocial behavior in Eastern and Western countries. Psychol Bull 2010;136:162–6; with permission.)

Are the effect sizes large enough to be considered important? Even small effect sizes can have large practical consequences. Because such a high percentage of children and adolescents spend large amounts of time playing violent games, small effects can accumulate and significantly influence individuals and society. In fact, the obtained effect sizes of violent video games on aggression-related variables are comparable in size with the effect of second-hand smoke on lung cancer and the effect of calcium intake on bone mass (see **Fig. 1**).[31]

Aggressive Cognition, Affect, and Behavior

Findings from experimental, correlational, and longitudinal studies generally show that violent video game play is a significant risk factor for aggression (**Box 2**). This effect has been demonstrated in both short-term and long-term contexts, and in diverse populations.

Studies suggest that violent video games increase aggression by increasing aggressive thoughts and emotions, even when their physiologic arousal properties have been controlled. Playing violent video games can prime aggressive thoughts, increase positive attitudes toward violence, and help create a hostile attribution bias: a tendency to perceive other people's behaviors as malevolent.[33–35] In the short term, exposure to video game violence produces feelings of anger and hostility in players.[36] Even the critics of violent game research support the findings on aggressive thoughts, arousal, and decreased prosocial behavior.[37] Over longer periods of time, such changes can lead to the development of an aggressive personality.[15]

Empathy, Desensitization, and Helping

Another line of research has found that video game violence produces desensitization to violence and decreases in empathy and helping. Desensitization can be defined as reduction in physiological and emotional reactivity to violence.[14] Short-term exposure to violent media has been shown to produce physiological desensitization in only 20 minutes, whereas habitual video game playing has been linked to chronic desensitization.[14,38,39]

A related line of research examined links between violent video games and empathy, the degree to which a person identifies and commiserates with a victim.[13]

Box 2
Effects of violent video games on aggressive behavior

- Experimental studies have been used to show causal effects of video game violence on immediate increases in aggression. For example, in a laboratory experiment, children and adolescents were more likely to blast a supposed opponent with loud noise through headphones after playing a violent video game compared with a nonviolent game.[17]

- Correlational studies enabled researchers to explore associations between violent video game play and real-life instances of aggression. For example, adolescents who had consumed greater amounts of video game violence were more likely to be involved in a physical fight.[32]

- Longitudinal studies have shown relationships between video game violence and increases of aggression over time. For example, children who played more violent games early in the school year were found to display more physical and verbal aggression 5 months later.[17]

- Meta-analyses combine results of multiple studies and provide the strongest evidence that video game violence increases the risk of aggression. The most recent meta-analysis in this area showed a significant effect of video game violence on aggressive behaviors across different types of research designs.[13]

Empathy has been shown to significantly mediate the link between violent video game play and aggressive behavior.[15] It seems that this emotional numbing can also lead to a reduction in helping behavior. For example, students who had just played a violent video game were less likely to perceive a fight they witnessed as serious or to help the injured victim.[16]

Attention Deficits and Cognitive Control

Findings of positive effects of gaming experience on visuospatial skills are sometimes misinterpreted to mean that video games benefit attention in general. However, a growing body of evidence suggests that video games may actually exacerbate attention problems and have harmful effects on some aspects of cognitive control.

- Several studies have found correlations between attention problems in childhood and video game play.[16,40,41] High excitement and rapid changes of focus that occur in many video games may weaken children's abilities to maintain focus on less exciting tasks (eg, schoolwork) and shorten their attention spans.
- In a longitudinal study on video game use and attention problems, video game play predicted children's attention problems 13 months later, even while controlling for other relevant variables (earlier attention problems, television viewing, and gender).[18] A 3-year longitudinal study of more than 3000 children found evidence of a bidirectional relation between attention problems and video game playing, and found a stronger relation between the amount of gaming and later attention problems than for the content of gaming.[42]
- Several studies have also shown negative relations between video game play and cognitive control.[43–45] It seems that video games have specific effects on different types of cognitive processing: they can increase visuospatial processing skills and can also harm proactive cognitive control.[27,45]

Video Game Addiction

There are now scores of studies looking at what is being called pathological gaming or video game "addiction." Many researchers define pathologic use of video games in the same way as pathological gambling, focusing on damage to family, social, school, occupational, and psychological functioning.[19] Like gambling, playing video games starts as a form entertainment. It becomes pathological for some people when video games start producing negative life consequences.[21] Overall, studies examining pathological video gaming show good reliability and validity. For example, a study conducted in the United States with a national sample of 1100 youth found that 8.5% of youth gamers could be classified as pathological,[21] and similar percentages are being found in other countries.[46–51] At present, video game addiction is not classified as a formal disorder in the *Diagnostic and Statistical Manual of Mental Disorders* (DSM). The American Psychiatric Association has proposed a new category for the DSM-V of addiction-like behavioral disorders. Gambling has been moved into this category, but more research is needed before video game and Internet addictions should be included.[52]

Video Games and School Performance

Several studies have found a significant negative relation between the amount of screen time (television viewing and video game play) and school performance of children, adolescents, and college students.[3,17,25,33,53,54] That is, high amounts of time on screen media are associated with poorer school performance. One explanation is the displacement hypothesis, which states that video games (and other screen media) may displace time that would otherwise be spent on activities such as reading, home-work,[32] There has been some evidence to support the displacement hypothesis. In one study of a large nationally represented sample of youth aged 10 to 19 years, gamers spent 30% less time reading and 34% less time doing homework in comparison with nongamers.[55]

POSITIVE EFFECTS OF VIDEO GAMES

Visual-Spatial Skills

Several studies show that video game play can improve a wide range of visual and spatial skills.[27–29,56]

- Correlational studies have found positive associations between gaming experi-ence and performance in numerous visual tasks, such as target localization[29] and faster visual reaction times.[8]
- Experimental studies have demonstrated that even as little as 10 hours of video game play can improve spatial attention and mental rotation.[27,57]

These beneficial effects may have a range of practical applications. For example, an early experimental study showed that Israeli Air Force cadets trained using the game *Space Fortress 2* had better subsequent flight performance.[58] As a result, the game became a part of the training program of the Israeli Air Force. The largest enhance-ments to visuospatial processing have been shown for fast-paced action games, which also often contain violence.[8] This fact illustrates the point that the effects of video games are not simple, and a game can simultaneously have positive effects (increased visuospatial skills) and negative effects (increased aggressive emotions, thoughts, and behaviors).

Educational Video Games

Video games are highly effective teachers. Well-designed video games are attention-grabbing, set clear objectives, provide feedback and reinforcement, actively involve the player, offer adaptable levels of difficulty, and use many other powerful teaching techniques.[20] A wide range of educational games have been developed, taking advan-tage of these features of video games and using them to teach specific knowledge and skills.

- Schools: Video games have been successfully used to teach children and adolescents a variety of topics, such as reading skills, mathematics, and biology.[9,59]
- Business: Video games are often used to teach job skills to employees. For example, Canon USA uses a video game to train copier technicians, Volvo uses an online game to teach car sales employees, and the US military uses video games to train combat skills and increase recruitment.[60,61]
- Health-related outcomes: Games have been developed to teach youth about smoking, diabetes, and cancer.[62–64] These games have been shown to be highly effective. For example, asthmatic children who played the game *Bronkie the Bronchiasaurus* showed significant improvements in their knowledge about asthma and self-care behaviors.[62]

Exergames

Video games have traditionally been a sedentary activity. However, in recent years a new type of video game has emerged that requires interactive physical activity. Exer-cise games, or exergames, combine video games and exercise.[65]

- Active games, such as *Dance Dance Revolution* and *Wii Fit* can increase energy expenditure, prolong time spent in physical activity, and increase preference for physical activity among players.[66–68]
- Exergames have been shown to increase engagement and enjoyment. For example, a 6-week-long training study demonstrated that interactive videobikes increase adherence to a training program and attitudes toward exercise compared with traditional bikes.[10]
- Particularly positive attitudes toward exergaming are found among sedentary individuals, indicating that this may be an effective way of increasing physical activity in this group.[65]

It is a worrying fact that American children tend to spend more than 6 hours per day watching television and playing video games, yet almost half of preschool children do not meet recommended levels of physical activity of at least 1 hour per day prescribed by the American Academy of Pediatrics.[3,69] Given the tremendous popularity of video games among youth, combining gaming and physical activity may be a good strategy to increase physical activity among children and adolescents.

Prosocial Video Games

Prosocial video games are those in which the primary purpose of the player is to help other game characters. Although the literature on the effects of prosocial games is much smaller than that on effects of violent video games, there is growing support for the idea that prosocial video games can promote prosocial tendencies.[11,70] It must be noted that games with violent content are not considered truly prosocial, even if the player's character is helping other players by killing mutual enemies.

Playing a nonviolent prosocial video game in the laboratory has actually been shown to decrease aggressive thoughts, feelings, and behaviors.[12,71] Prosocial video game play can also increase prosocial thoughts, enhance empathy, and promote helping behavior.[70,72–74] For example, in a series of experimental studies, playing a prosocial video game made participants more predisposed to help the researcher pick up fallen pencils, agree to participate in further experiments, and come to the aid of a female experimenter who was being harassed by a supposed ex-boyfriend (actually a confederate).[11]

These findings are not limited to laboratory experiments. For example, a large-sample correlational study showed significant associations between prosocial video game play and prosocial behaviors in real life (eg, spending money to help those who are in need).[71] In a follow-up longitudinal study, prosocial game play predicted increases in prosocial behavior among children over a period of 3 to 4 months, confirming that prosocial games can have a long-term impact on helping.[12]

GUIDELINES FOR PARENTS, PEDIATRICIANS, AND OTHER CAREGIVERS

The research on positive and negative effects of video games clearly shows that video games are effective teachers that can affect players in multiple ways simultaneously. Therefore, the original question asked about whether games were "good" or "bad" is demonstrated to be a false dichotomy. Some effects are harmful (such as effects of violent video games on aggression and the effect of screen time on poorer school performance), whereas others are beneficial (eg, effects of action games on visual-spatial skills).

Suggestions are made in **Box 3** as to what can be done to maximize the positive effects of video game use and minimize harm.

Box 3

Advice for pediatricians, parents, and other caregivers on choosing and using video games

- Ask about games and other media use at well-child checkups. Pediatricians and general practitioners are in the unique role of helping parents to understand that they need to take their children's media use seriously. Parents setting limits on the amount and content of children's media is a powerful protective factor for children.[2,17,32]

- Do not rely solely on ratings. Even games rated E for Everyone often contain depictions of violence.[75] Instead, try playing the game yourself, ask someone to demonstrate it for you, or look for descriptions or video clips of the game on the Internet.

- Choose well. Select nonviolent games that have been shown to have positive effects, such as educational games, prosocial games, and exergames. Do not allow access to violent video games, defined as games in which you must harm other characters to advance.

- Set limits on both the amount and content of games. Create clear rules about amount of time and the kind of content that is allowed. Even positive games can be played too much. The American Academy of Pediatrics recommends no more than 1 to 2 hours of total screen time (video games, TV, DVDs, computer, and so forth, all summed together) per day.

- Keep game devices in public space. When gaming devices are in private space (child's bedroom), it is very difficult to control either content or time. Move them to public space (eg, living room, kitchen).

- Stay involved. Explain to your children why playing violent games or playing games for an excessive amount of time may be harmful to them. Discuss your family's values concerning violence and aggression. Help them learn to make good choices.

- Spread the word. Help educate others in your community (parents, youth, public officials). Although almost 100% of pediatricians have been convinced by the data that the media have significant effects,[76] the public do not know this. The mainstream media often sensationalize and polarize discussion on this topic; it is important that people understand that there are both potential benefits and harms to be derived from game play.

REFERENCES

1. Gentile DA. Pathological video-game use among youth ages 8-18: a national study. Psychol Sci 2009;20(5):594–602.
2. Gentile DA, Walsh DA. A normative study of family media habits. J Appl Dev Psychol 2002;23:157–78.
3. Rideout VJ, Foehr UG, Roberts DF. Generation M^2—media in the lives of 8- to 18-year olds. Menlo Park (CA): Kaiser Family Foundation; 2010.
4. Bailey K, West R, Anderson CA. The influence of video games on social, cognitive, and affective information processing. In: Decety J, Cacioppo J, editors. Handbook of social neuroscience. New York: Oxford University Press; 2011. p. 1001–11.
5. Cavalli E. Jack Thompson reaches out to Take-Two exec's mother. Wired; 2008. Available at: http://www.wired.com/gamelife/2008/04/jack-thompson-p/. Accessed January 2, 2012.
6. Entertainment Software Association. The transformation of the video game industry. ESA; 2011. Available at: http://www.theesa.com/games-improving-what-matters/ESA_FS_Transformation_2011.pdf. Accessed January 2, 2012.
7. Entertainment Software Association. Essential facts about games and violence. ESA; 2011. Available at: http://www.theesa.com/facts/pdfs/ESA_EF_About_Games_and_Violence.pdf. Accessed January 2, 2012.

8. Achtman RL, Green CS, Bavelier D. Video games as a tool to train visual skills. Restor Neurol Neurosci 2008;26(4–5):435–46.
9. Murphy R, Penuel W, Means B, et al. E-DESK: a review of recent evidence on the effectiveness of discrete educational software. Menlo Park (CA): SRI International; 2001.
10. Rhodes RE, Warburton DE, Bredin SS. Predicting the effect of interactive video bikes on exercise adherence: an efficacy trial. Psychol Health Med 2009;14(6): 631–40.
11. Greitemeyer T, Osswald S. Effects of prosocial video games on prosocial behavior. J Pers Soc Psychol 2010;98(2):211–21.
12. Sestir MA, Bartholow BD. Violent and nonviolent video games produce opposing effects on aggressive and prosocial outcomes. J Exp Soc Psychol 2010;46:934–42.
13. Anderson CA, Shibuya A, Ihori N, et al. Violent video game effects on aggression, empathy, and prosocial behavior in Eastern and Western countries. Psychol Bull 2010;136:151–73.
14. Carnagey NL, Anderson CA, Bushman BJ. The effect of video game violence on physiological desensitization to real-life violence. J Exp Soc Psychol 2007;43:489–96.
15. Bartholow BD, Sestir MA, Davis E. Correlates and consequences of exposure to video game violence: hostile personality, empathy, and aggressive behavior. Psychol Bull 2005;31:1573–86.
16. Bushman BJ, Anderson CA. Comfortably numb: desensitizing effects of violent media on helping others. Psychol Sci 2009;20:273–7.
17. Anderson CA, Gentile DA, Buckley KE. Violent video game effects on children and adolescents: theory, research, and public policy. New York: Oxford University Press; 2007.
18. Swing EL, Gentile DA, Anderson CA, et al. Television and video game exposure and the development of attention problems. Pediatrics 2010;126:214–21.
19. Anderson CA, Gentile DA, Dill KE. Prosocial, antisocial and other effects of recreational video games. In: Singer DG, Singer JL, editors. Handbook of children and the media. 2nd edition. Thousand Oaks (CA): Sage; 2012. p. 231–72.
20. Gentile DA, Gentile JR. Violent video games as exemplary teachers: a conceptual analysis. J Youth Adolesc 2008;9:127–41.
21. Gentile DA. The multiple dimensions of video game effects. Child Dev Perspect 2011;5:75–81.
22. Gentile DA, Stone W. Violent video game effects on children and adolescents: a review of the literature. Minerva Pediatr 2005;57:337–58.
23. Khoo A, Gentile DA. Problem based learning in the world of games. In: Tan OS, Hung D, editors. Problem-based learning and e-learning breakthroughs. Singapore: Thomson Publishing; 2007. p. 97–129.
24. Berkey CS, Rockett HRH, Field AE, et al. Activity, dietary intake, and weight changes in a longitudinal study of preadolescent and adolescent boys and girls. Pediatrics 2000;105:e56.
25. Cordes C, Miller E. Fool's gold: a critical look at computers in childhood. College Park (MD): Alliance for Childhood; 2000.
26. Hamalainen R. Designing and evaluating collaboration in a virtual game environment for vocational learning. Comput Educ 2008;50:98–109.
27. Green CS, Bavelier D. Action video game modifies visual selective attention. Nature 2003;423(6939):534–7.
28. Green CS, Bavelier D. Effect of action video games on the spatial distribution of visuospatial attention. J Exp Psychol Hum Percept Perform 2006;32(6): 1465–78.

29. Green CS, Bavelier D. Action video game experience alters the spatial resolution of attention. Psychol Sci 2007;18(1):88–94.
30. Deutsch JE, Borbely M, Filler J, et al. Use of a low-cost, commercially available gaming console (Wii) for rehabilitation of an adolescent with cerebral palsy. Phys Ther 2008;8:1196–207.
31. Bushman BJ, Huesmann LR. Effects of televised violence on aggression. In: Singer D, Singer J, editors. Handbook of children and the media. Thousand Oaks (CA): Sage Publications; 2001. p. 223–54.
32. Gentile DA, Lynch PJ, Linder JR, et al. The effects of violent video game habits on adolescent hostility, aggressive behaviors, and school performance. J Adolesc 2004;27(1):5–22.
33. Anderson CA, Dill KE. Video games and aggressive thoughts, feelings, and behavior in the laboratory and in life. J Pers Soc Psychol 2000;78:772–90.
34. Funk JB, Baldacci HB, Pasold T, et al. Violence exposure in real-life, video games, television, movies, and the Internet: is there desensitization? J Adolesc 2004;27(1):23–39.
35. Kirsh SJ. Seeing the world through "Mortal Kombat" colored glasses: violent video games and the development of a short-term hostile attribution bias. Childhood 1998;5:177–84. Available at: http://chd.sagepub.com/content/5/2/177.abstract. Accessed March 16, 2012.
36. Carnagey NL, Anderson CA. The effects of reward and punishment in violent video games on aggressive affect, cognition, and behavior. Psychol Sci 2005; 16:882–9.
37. Ferguson CJ. Evidence for publication bias in video game violence effects literature: a meta-analytic review. Aggression and Violent Behaviour 2007;12:470–82.
38. Bailey K, West R, Anderson CA. The association between chronic exposure to video game violence and affective picture processing: an ERP study. Cogn Affect Behav Neurosci 2011;11:259–76.
39. Bartholow BD, Bushman BJ, Sestir MA. Chronic violent video game exposure and desensitization to violence: behavioral and event-related brain potential data. J Exp Soc Psychol 2005;42(2):283–90.
40. Bioulac S, Arfi L, Bouvard MP. Attention deficit/hyperactivity disorder and video games: a comparative study of hyperactive and control children. Eur Psychiatry 2008;23(2):134–41.
41. Mistry KB, Minkovitz CS, Strobino DM, et al. Children's television exposure and behavioral and social outcomes at 5.5 years: does timing of exposure matter? Pediatrics 2007;120:762–9.
42. Gentile DA, Swing EL, Lim CG, et al. Video game playing, attention problems, and impulsiveness: evidence of bidirectional causality. Psychology of Popular Media Culture 2012;1:62–70.
43. Bailey K, West R, Anderson CA. A negative association between video game experience and proactive cognitive control. Psychophysiology 2010;47:34–42.
44. Kronenberger WG, Mathews VP, Dunn DW, et al. Media violence exposure and executive functioning in aggressive and control adolescents. J Clin Psychol 2005;61(6):725–37.
45. Mathews VP, Kronenberger WG, Wang Y, et al. Media violence exposure and frontal lobe activation measured by functional magnetic resonance imaging in aggressive and nonaggressive adolescents. J Comput Assist Tomogr 2005;29:287–92.
46. Choo H, Gentile DA, Sim T, et al. Pathological video-gaming among Singaporean youth. Ann Acad Med Singapore 2010;39:822–9.

47. Gentile DA, Choo H, Liau A, et al. Pathological video game use among youth: a two-year longitudinal study. Pediatrics 2011;127:e319–29.

48. Peng LH, Li X. A survey of Chinese college students addicted to video games. China Education Innovation Herald 2009;28:111–2.

49. Porter G, Starcevic V, Berle D, et al. Recognizing problem video game use. Aust N Z J Psychiatry 2010;44:120–8.

50. Grüsser SM, Thalemann R, Griffiths MD. Excessive computer game playing: evidence for addiction and aggression? Cyberpsychol Behav 2007;10(2):290–2.

51. Ko CH, Yen JY, Yen CF, et al. Factors predictive for incidence and remission of Internet addiction in young adolescents: a prospective study. Cyberpsychol Behav 2007;10(4):545–51.

52. APA. DSM-V development. American Psychiatric Association; 2012. Available at: http://www.dsm5.org/Pages/Default.aspx. Accessed January 2, 2012.

53. Chan PA, Rabinowitz T. A cross-sectional analysis of video games and attention deficit hyperactivity disorder symptoms in adolescents. Ann Gen Psychiatr 2006;5:16.

54. Sharif I, Sargent JD. Association between television, movie, and video game exposure and school performance. Pediatrics 2006;118(4):1061–70.

55. Cummings HMM, Vandewater EAP. Relation of adolescent video game play to time spent in other activities. Arch Pediatr Adolesc Med 2007;161(7):684–9.

56. Dye MW, Green CS, Bavelier D. The development of attention skills in action video game players. Neuropsychologia 2009;47(8–9):1780–9.

57. Feng J, Spence I, Pratt J. Playing an action video game reduces gender differences in spatial cognition. Psychol Sci 2007;18(10):850–5.

58. Gopher D, Weil M, Bareket T. Transfer of skill from a computer game trainer to flight. Hum Factors 1994;36:1–19.

59. Corbett AT, Koedinger KR, Hadley W. Cognitive tutors: from the research classroom to all classrooms. In: Goodman PS, editor. Technology enhanced learning. Mahwah (NJ): Lawrence Erlbaum; 2001. p. 235–63.

60. Entertainment Software Association. Games: improving education. Available at: http://www.theesa.com/games-improving-what-matters/ESA_FS_Education_2011.pdf. Accessed January 2, 2012.

61. Flood S. All play and more work. In: Computing. 2006. Available at: http://www.computing.co.uk/computing/analysis/2152597/play-work. Accessed January 2, 2012.

62. Lieberman DA. Management of chronic pediatric diseases with interactive health games: Theory and research findings. J Ambul Care Manage 2001;24(1):26–38.

63. Brown SJ, Lieberman DA, Gemeny BA, et al. Educational video game for juvenile diabetes: results of a controlled trial. Med Inform 1997;22(1):77–89.

64. Kato PM, Cole SW, Bradlyn AS, et al. A video game improves behavioral outcomes in adolescents and young adults with cancer: a randomized trial. Pediatrics 2008;122:e305–17.

65. Klein MJ, Simmers CS. Exergaming: virtual inspiration, real perspiration. Young Consumers 2009;10:35–45.

66. Biddiss E, Irwin J. Active video games to promote physical activity in children and youth. Arch Pediatr Adolesc Med 2010;164(7):664–72.

67. Graf DL, Pratt LV, Hester CN, et al. Playing active video games increases energy expenditure in children. Pediatrics 2009;124(2):534–40.

68. Mellecker RR, McManus AM. Energy expenditure and cardiovascular responses to seated and active gaming in children. Arch Pediatr Adolesc Med 2008;162(9):886–91.

69. Tucker P. The physical activity levels of preschool-aged children: a systematic review. Early Child Res Q 2008;3(4):547–58.
70. Gentile DA, Anderson CA, Yukawa S, et al. The effects of prosocial video games on prosocial behaviors: international evidence from correlational, longitudinal, and experimental studies. Pers Soc Psychol Bull 2009;35(6):752–63.
71. Narvaez D, Mattan B, MacMichael C, et al. Kill bandits, collect gold or save the dying: the effects of playing a prosocial video game. Media Psychology Review 2008;1(1). Available at: http://mprcenter.org/mpr/index.php?option=com_content&view=article&id=35&Itemid=121. Accessed.
72. Greitemeyer T, Osswald S. Prosocial video games reduce aggressive cognitions. J Exp Soc Psychol 2009;4:896–900.
73. Greitemeyer T, Osswald S. Playing prosocial video games increases the accessibility of prosocial thoughts. J Soc Psychol 2011;151(2):121–8.
74. Greitemeyer T, Osswald S, Brauer M. Playing prosocial video games increases empathy and decreases schadenfreude. Emotion 2010;10(6):796–802.
75. Gentile DA. The rating systems for media products. In: Calvert S, Wilson B, editors. Handbook of children, media, and development. Oxford (United Kingdom): Blackwell Publishing; 2008. p. 527–51.
76. Gentile DA, Oberg C, Sherwood NE, et al. Well-child exams in the video age: pediatricians and the AAP guidelines for children's media use. Pediatrics 2004; 114:1235–41.

The New Threat of Digital Marketing

Kathryn C. Montgomery, PhD[a],*, Jeff Chester, MSW[b],
Sonya A. Grier, MBA, PhD[c], Lori Dorfman, DrPH[d]

KEYWORDS

- Marketing • Advertising • Childhood obesity • Policy • Digital media • Social media

KEY POINTS

- Today's children and teens are growing up in a ubiquitous digital media environment, in which mobile devices, instant messaging, social networks, virtual reality, avatars, interactive games, and online video have become ingrained in their personal and social experiences.
- A large infrastructure of market research firms, advertising agencies, trend analysis companies, and digital strategists is continually monitoring how children and teens engage with new media.
- The exploding popularity of social media and the emergence of marketing strategies designed for those popular networks have made young people particularly vulnerable to interactive advertising.
- The rise of smartphones and elaborate mobile marketing campaigns has proved especially effective in reaching young people, as have interactive games and other immersive media.
- In the hands of fast-food, snack-food, and soft drink companies that target children and adolescents, the new marketing landscape raises particularly critical issues in light of the current obesity crisis.

In 2009, McDonald's collaborated with the blockbuster movie *Avatar* on an elaborate multiplatform cross-promotion campaign designed to "drive mass awareness and traffic" to its fast-food restaurants around the world.[1] The campaign incorporated a variety of touchpoints—including television, restaurant displays, packaging, toys,

This article was supported by the Robert Wood Johnson Foundation Healthy Eating Research initiative as well as the National Policy & Legal Analysis Network to Prevent Childhood Obesity for supporting the research for this article.
[a] School of Communication, American University, 4400 Massachusetts Avenue, NW, Washington, DC 20016, USA; [b] Center for Digital Democracy, 1621 Connecticut Avenue, NW, Suite 550, Washington, DC 20009, USA; [c] Department of Marketing, Kogod School of Business, American University, 4400 Massachusetts Avenue, NW, Washington, DC 20016, USA; [d] Berkeley Media Studies Group, 2130 Center Street, Suite 302, Berkeley, CA 94704, USA
* Corresponding author.
E-mail address: kcm@american.edu

Pediatr Clin N Am 59 (2012) 659–675
doi:10.1016/j.pcl.2012.03.022
0031-3955/12/$ – see front matter © 2012 Elsevier Inc. All rights reserved.

pediatric.theclinics.com

and social media—designed to reach and engage young people throughout the contemporary media landscape.[2] At the heart of the campaign, according to McDonald's, was "an immersive digital experience centered around Pandora, the mythical planet of *Avatar*," whose purpose was to "immerse you in an extraordinary, technology-driven journey that's sure to 'Thrill the Senses'."[3] Avatar "Thrill Cards" on Big Mac packages could be placed in front of a Webcam or cell phone camera to activate McDonald's-branded McD Vision software, enabling users to enter the virtual Pandora-themed online worlds and play an interactive Pandora Quest game. Codes placed in Happy Meal toys gave children access to special features on the Web site, an effort designed to further integrate their offline and online experiences for marketing purposes.[4] The goal of the campaign was to drive "deeper engagement with the brand," ultimately leading to "repeat purchases of iconic products, such as the Big Mac."[2]

In many ways, the *Avatar* campaign represents an extension of McDonald's long-established pattern of marketing through movie cross-promotions and toy tie-ins, a practice that has raised concerns from public health experts and advocacy groups.[5] As these campaigns have moved further into the digital realm, however, they have morphed into something distinctly different. The forms of advertising and marketing to children through new media depart in significant ways from the more familiar commercial advertising and promotion in children's television.[6] Today's contemporary marketing efforts are increasingly multidimensional—simultaneously and purposefully integrated into a range of social media and online applications: Facebook, Twitter, YouTube, gaming, and mobile communications.

The interactive media are ushering in an entirely new set of relationships, breaking down the traditional barriers between content and commerce and creating unprecedented intimacies between children and marketers. Unlike television, where children's exposure to commercials is limited to brief intervals during the times when they are viewing the programs, digital marketing is now woven into the fabric of young people's daily experiences, integrated not only into their media content but also into their social and personal relationships. Young people are not just viewing content but also inhabiting media environments where entertainment, communication, and marketing are combined in a seamless stream of compelling sounds and images.

These trends have significant implications for young peoples' health and well-being. Parents, health professionals, and policy makers need to understand the changing nature of marketing in the digital era, how it differs from traditional forms of advertising directed at children, and how it is influencing young people's behaviors. Marketers are developing and implementing a new generation of marketing techniques, many of which operate below the level of parental or public awareness and push the boundaries of appropriateness.

This article provides a brief overview of the growing digital media and marketing landscape, focusing on 4 important developments that are shaping marketing strategies and techniques. It highlights techniques that are used by fast-food, snack-food, and soft drink companies to target children and adolescents, which raise particularly critical issues in light of the current obesity crisis. The trends and practices discussed, however, are emblematic of a paradigm shift in contemporary global advertising and are used by a wide variety companies, promoting not only food and beverages but also toys, clothing, entertainment, and brands popular with young people.[7,8] Several important issues raised by these developments that require further study are identified and current policy developments aimed at addressing some of the emerging digital marketing practices are highlighted.

THE EXPANDING MEDIA AND MARKETING LANDSCAPE

Today's children and teens are growing up in a ubiquitous digital media environment, in which mobile devices, instant messaging, social networks, virtual reality, avatars, interactive games, and online video have become ingrained in their personal and social experiences. Members of this generation of young people are, in many ways, living their lives online. Several factors—the growth of the Internet, the proliferation of digital media platforms and content, and, in particular, the rapid penetration of mobile phones—have triggered a jump in media time for children and teens.

According to a 2010 study by the Kaiser Family Foundation, young people now spend more than 7.5 hours daily consuming media. When multitasking behaviors are included, this means that today's youth "pack a total of 10 hours and 45 minutes worth of media content into those daily 7.5 hours national average—an increase of almost 2¼ hours of media exposure per day over the past five years."[9] The increase in media consumption has been the most significant among African American and Hispanic youth, who have approximately 5 more hours of media exposure per day than the aforementioned national average for youth. These differences remain even after statistical controls are included for other demographic factors, such as age, parent education, or whether a child is from a single-parent or two-parent family.[9]

Marketers seek not simply to expose young people to ads but to foster ongoing engagement—by encouraging them to interact with, befriend, and integrate brands into their personal identities and social worlds.[10–13] In some cases, this includes offering incentives to encourage youth to participate in developing new products, designing packages, and creating online advertising that they then distribute among their friends.

The digital marketplace is undergoing rapid innovation as new technologies and software applications continue to reshape the media landscape and user behaviors. Four major developments are particularly critical in the growing arsenal of tools used by companies targeting children and teens: (1) the growth of interactive games and increasing sophistication of augmented reality and other immersive features of digital media, (2) the rapid explosion of social media and the emergence of marketing strategies designed for those popular platforms, (3) the further development and proliferation of data collection and profiling techniques, and (4) the rise of smartphones and mobile marketing. In each of these areas, companies are harnessing a new generation of marketing techniques to reach and influence young people.

Using Web analytics, conversation targeting, and other new forms of digital surveillance, marketers can now track individuals—including youth—online, across media, and in the real world, monitoring their interactions, social relationships, and locations. Increasingly, these various forms of analysis can take place in real time, following users' movements and behaviors from moment to moment and in the process assessing their reactions to marketing techniques. As a result, marketing messages can be tested, refined, and tailored for maximum effect.[14,15]

A large infrastructure of market research firms, advertising agencies, trend analysis companies, and digital strategists is continually monitoring how children and teens engage with new media.[16–19] Market researchers use the expertise of an increasingly diverse array of specialists in sociology, anthropology, psychology, and neuroscience to explore youth subcultures and conduct motivational research.[18] A considerable amount of contemporary market research is focused on identifying ways to tap into the critical developmental stages of childhood and adolescence. Researchers are tracking how young people are integrating digital technologies into their lives and identifying social and psychographic subcategories based on sophisticated new data gathering and data analysis techniques.[20–22]

Marketers are not just tapping into these new patterns but also actively cultivating and promoting them to foster ongoing relationships and ubiquitous connectivity with brands. Digital campaigns can be highly complex, combining mobile, online video, interactive television, and social networks and creating a powerful multiplier effect by spreading messages extensively throughout and among social groups.[23,24] Major media companies are now offering cross-platform marketing opportunities, where, in a single buy, advertisers can target customers across a company's media properties, online and offline. Increasing consolidation within the entertainment media, advertising, and technology fields further enhances the ability of companies to deploy a variety of advertising and brand promotion strategies across a wide spectrum of media properties so that connections to brands are uninterrupted.[23,25]

Children and teenagers continue to be a lucrative market for advertisers, with advertising time on TV and new media platforms generating record sales.[26] Young people between the ages of 8 and 15 control over $40 billion in spending annually. Children are also using new media technologies at an earlier age and spending increasing amounts of time engaged in an expanding array of new platforms, including virtual worlds, interactive games, and mobile apps. As *Adweek* reported, "80% of kids under the age of 5 use the Internet weekly, and 60% of kids 3 and younger are now watching videos online."[27] Approximately 10% of 6 to 8 years olds, 23% of 9 to 10 year olds, and 41% of children ages 11 to 12 are social network users, according to eMarketer.[28] Today, by age 11, "half of kids have cell phones," according to research released this year by LMX Family/Ipsos OTX. That same report, explained *Advertising Age,* noted that "pre-schoolers [are] adopting digital habits or being exposed to new devices even faster than tweens, a sign of the speed with which digital technology is reshaping media and marketing habits for the youngest children."[29] As discussed later, teens are among the most active users of cell phones for a variety of applications, including text messaging and video.

SOCIAL MEDIA MARKETING

Online social networks are among the most popular digital media platforms for young people, with more than three-fourths of US online youth ages 12 to 17 participating in them.[30,31] Social media resonate strongly with many of the fundamental developmental tasks of childhood and adolescence, such as identity exploration, social interaction, and autonomy. They provide an accessible, user-friendly template for creating and expressing a public and private persona in cyberspace.[32,33] Many teens rely on social networks to seek help for their personal problems, explore their own sexual identities, find support groups for handling emotional crises in their lives, and sometimes talk about things they do not feel comfortable or safe discussing with their own parents.[34]

Social media platforms provide digital marketers with a palette of new interactive techniques.[35–37] They give marketers access to the relationships among individuals and communities in ways never before possible. Marketers routinely monitor and tap into what is known as the *social graph*, the complex web of relationships among individuals facilitated and tracked online.[38] Using a host of new techniques and measurement tools, social media marketers can know the breadth and depth of these online social relationships as well as how they function, understanding who influences whom, and how the process of influence works. Social media marketers can now—on an almost second-by-second basis—track and analyze the online behaviors and expressions of consumers, including individuals or sources of greatest peer influence.

By its nature, social media marketing is designed to facilitate, accelerate, and in many ways automate the process of brand or product endorsement among young people whose lives and social interactions are linked and monitored online. Viral marketing is a core principle of social media advertising. By tapping into the online social graph, marketers can orchestrate elaborate, instantaneous viral marketing campaigns, identifying individuals who are most likely to create their own user-generated marketing messages among their wide circle of social relationships and providing incentives to encourage brand promotion. Social media marketers use a variety of incentives, such as contests, prizes, and free products, to encourage individuals to create and promote ads that are distributed among friends and acquaintances online. The practice is expanding to an array of new platforms—including blogs, mobile phones, and online video and games. For example, PepsiCo's Mountain Dew DEWmocracy campaign used Facebook and other social networking platforms to create a multilayered effort combining a variety of digital techniques. Users and fans of the brand were invited to participate in a crowd-sourcing project to come up with names for new versions of the popular soft drink and vote on the best ones.[39]

Marketers have developed strategies to take advantage of the special relationship between young people and social networks. An entire infrastructure has emerged—from specialty advertising agencies to tracking and measurement services to third-party developers—to facilitate social media marketing. Spending for such marketing was predicted to reach $10.3 billion in 2011, up 41.4% from $7.3 billion in 2010. By 2015, social media spending is expected to reach $29.1 billion.[40–42]

DATA COLLECTION AND BEHAVIORAL TARGETING

Data collection is at the core of contemporary digital marketing; individual consumers are tagged with unique identifiers when they engage with online services, and then tracked, profiled, and interactively targeted for personalized marketing and advertising as they navigate the Web.[15] Advertisers and marketers have developed an array of sophisticated and ever-evolving data collection and profiling applications, honed from the latest developments in such fields as semantics, artificial intelligence, auction theory, social network analysis, data mining, and statistical modeling. Powerful analytical software mines data from Internet, Web, and social media applications, identifying patterns of user behavior to help craft and refine marketing strategies.

Growing investments in online marketing and data collection companies are expanding the field's capacity to deliver advertising based on harvesting individual users' online data.[43,44] Vast amounts of user data are now regularly mined and stored in behavioral targeting warehouses and other databases—and used in an instant to update online targeting profiles.[45] Individual consumers are being bought and sold via online advertising exchanges and other services so they can be targeted with interactive advertising.[46]

Youth can be lured to any site for advertising targeting using video, music, or other applications.[47] Data are collected online from youth through a variety of techniques. For example, contests, sweepstakes, "free" offers, and "point" schemes can deliver detailed information on particular users (name, address, e-mail address, cell phone number, and so forth). Immersive interactive applications, such as games, online video, and so-called rich media, are often designed to engage in data capture—including personal details as well as user-response metrics.

Passive data collection, through the use of cookies, IP addresses, and other data that the industry considers nonpersonally identifiable, enables marketers to effectively track and target individual users. Increasingly, data collection and targeting are not restricted to individual Web sites but are able to follow individuals across the Web and on mobile phones. In many cases, behavioral and other information that have become part of a person's profile can be sold to third parties, without an individual's knowledge or consent.

In 2009, the *Wall Street Journal* conducted an investigation of 50 Web sites popular with US children and teens, discovering that more than 4000 cookies, beacons, and other pieces of tracking technology were placed on the computers of those who visited the sites. "Marketers are spying more on young Internet users than on their parents, building detailed profiles of their activities and interests," the *Journal* found. Eight of the Web sites in the survey were owned by Viacom's Nickelodeon, and an average of 81 tracking tools were installed on the computers that accessed those sites.[48,49] Another study found that approximately half of the leading children's online sites engaged in forms of behavioral profiling, and most sites tracked a child's actions on Web sites.[50]

MOBILE MARKETING

Mobile and location marketing are quickly reshaping the entire advertising landscape. Mobile devices are nearly ubiquitous; smartphones enable access to a rich array of Internet applications, including those taking advantage of global positioning systems; local advertisers have new, inexpensive tools to deliver advertisements on mobile phones and in stores; and social networks are expanding their enterprises into the mobile arena through ventures, such as FourSquare, Gowalla, and Facebook's own location-based services.[51] Mobile video provides marketers with the ability to target advertising formatted for devices and users with increasing precision and offers a variety of formats to promote brands, collect data, and drive viral messaging.[52,53]

Smartphones that provide for ready Internet access and deliver multimedia services account for 40% of mobile phone subscriptions in the United States and were predicted to become the dominant type of cell phone by the end of 2011.[54,55] Many lower-income consumers use their mobile phones instead of traditional landlines, and many of these phones have some form of Internet access.[56] Mobile phone use has risen dramatically among children and teens. As a 2010 Kaiser Family Foundation study noted, "Over the past five years, there has been a huge increase in [cell phone] ownership among 8- to 18-year-olds: from 39% to 66%.... During this period, cell phones... have become true multi-media devices: in fact, young people now spend more time listening to music, playing games, and watching TV on their cell phones (a total of :49 daily) than they spend talking on them (:33)."[57]

Children ages 6 to 12 use their cell phones to surf the Internet, download applications, update their social networks, and send and receive text messages.[58] Nielsen reported, "Children begin downloading apps on a parents' phone at an average age of 9 years old," and parents explained, "30% of the apps on their phones were installed by their kids."[59] Children of color are particularly avid users of mobile and other new technologies.[60] As a recent study explained, when African American and Hispanic children own mobile phones, they "spend more time talking, texting and using media on cell phones than white children."[61] Lower-income black and Hispanic children, the study notes, "consume more digital media overall than their higher-income white peers."[61,62]

Teens remain quintessential early adopters in their use of mobile phones, avidly embracing a variety of Web applications and communication tools. Nielsen reports that teens ages 13 to 17 watch more video via their phones than any other group (approximately 7 hours and 13 minutes per month each, on average, compared with the next highest group—18–24 year olds—who averaged 4 hours and 20 minutes per month during the second quarter of 2010).[63] Text messaging has grown dramatically among teens, who "on average [are] sending or receiving 3339 texts a month," according to the Nielsen Company. "No one texts more than teens (ages 13–17)," adds Nielsen, with female and male teens averaging 753 minutes and 535 minutes a month, respectively.[64]

Mobile marketing techniques have been designed to harness the rich interactivity available on a small screen, incorporating a range of different direct-response actions and taking advantage of impulsivity, social connectivity, communications, and location. This approach also reflects and supports emerging styles of consumption behaviors, such as collaborative consumption. For example, applications have been created that enable a mobile user to connect seamlessly to a brand message through several special brand units that allow engaging in click to call, click to video, click to SMS, and so forth.[65] These new interactive, call-to-action formats foster instantaneous results, such as the delivery of mobile coupons through text messaging, scanning barcodes, or clicking on banner advertisements. Mobile landing pages—Web sites designed specifically for mobile Internet use—can be designed (via testing) to facilitate the desired brand responses. An array of methods to measure how users interact with mobile campaigns is used to assess their effectiveness.[65–67]

Mobile apps have enjoyed spectacular popularity in recent years, with more than 300,000 new apps appearing between 2008 and 2010 and more than 10.9 billion downloads worldwide in 2010 alone. According to one industry estimate, global app downloads will reach 76.9 billion in 2014, with revenues approaching $35 billion.[68] Many of these applications will be either advertising supported or advertising related.[60] For example, the location-based game MyTown, which gives points for checking in at stores, reported that quick-service restaurant chains (including Subway, McDonald's, Burger King, Taco Bell, Pizza Hut, Domino's Pizza, and Wendy's) made up 8 of the top 10 places favored by its users.[69]

With the phenomenal growth of mobile technologies and their rapid integration into young peoples' lives, mobile marketing has grown exponentially during a short period of time. The ubiquity of mobile phones gives marketers unprecedented ability to follow young people throughout their daily lives, delivering highly enticing marketing offers that are designed to trigger impulsive behaviors and linking point-of-influence techniques to point-of-purchase opportunities, thus short-circuiting the possibility of reflection or deliberation.

These powerful and intense forms of digital marketing are also completely integrated into teen social relationships and daily, minute-by-minute communications, adding the element of peer influence to what is already a powerful combination of multiple marketing appeals. Mobile marketing has also brought a convergence of other problematic techniques: offering a steady stream of immersive environments through video and interactive games; extending Facebook and other social networks onto a new, ever-present platform; and merging sophisticated data collection and behavioral profiling techniques with location tracking and path-to-purchase metrics.[70]

INTERACTIVE GAMES AND IMMERSIVE ENVIRONMENTS

Interactive games remain one of the fastest-growing forms of entertainment, surpassing even movie box offices in earnings, with revenues expected to reach $24.8 billion by 2013.[71,72] Gaming has evolved from a small pool of computer-based games into a multi-platform phenomenon, operating not only on PCs and mobile devices but also on dedicated consoles (eg, Nintendo Wii and Microsoft Xbox), which now constitute more than 25% of all online gaming.[73] According to a recent Kaiser Family Foundation study, video game playing has increased significantly over the past 5 years, primarily because of an increase in cell phone and handheld playing. Sixty percent of young people play video games. Hispanic and African Americans are particularly avid game players, spending significantly more time with them than white youth.[9]

Interactive video games are prime examples of the increasingly immersive nature of digital media. Recent innovations, such as augmented reality, which deliberately blurs the lines between the real world and the virtual world, have made games even more compelling, intense, and realistic. Through the use of state-of-the-art animation, high-definition video, and augmented reality, immersive environments can create a 3-D experience, surrounding and engrossing a person with powerful, realistic images and sounds and fostering a subjective feeling of being inside the action, a mental state that is frequently accompanied, in the words of writer and game designer Allen Varney, by "intense focus, loss of self, distorted time sense, effortless action."[74] Interactive video games and other immersive environments can also induce a state of flow, causing individuals to lose any sense of the passage of time.[75]

Marketers have seized on the immersive properties in interactive games to promote their brands to young people. In-game advertising has its roots in a long marketing tradition of product placement in movies and television, with brands paying or otherwise providing compensation to producers and directors who agree to insert a product or logo into their storylines. With the growing popularity of video games, the practice was adapted for that environment and has grown increasingly sophisticated. Advertising can be incorporated into a game's storyline and programmed to respond to player actions in real time, changing, adding, or updating messages to tailor their appeal to particular individuals.[76,77] Technological innovations are turning gaming into fully engaging, immersive experiences, and advertising-connected games are available on multiple platforms, including game consoles, personal computers, and mobile devices.

Immersive marketing techniques routinely integrate advertising and content in such a way as to make the two indistinguishable.[78–80] Marketers can seamlessly incorporate brands into the flow of the immersive experience, using a highly sophisticated, finely tuned strategy that combines product placement, behavioral targeting, and viral marketing to foster deep, ongoing relationships between brands and individuals. Digital marketers have perfected software for tracking consumer behavior in video games as well as other interactive platforms.[81–83] These techniques enable marketers to create particularly intense experiences, plunging users into the center of the action through the use of avatars or first-person shooter devices that induce a strong sense of subjectivity and heighten emotional arousal. The combination of all these elements creates an experience that is designed to extend engagement with the game—and the brand—over long periods of time.

Such marketing techniques may be particularly challenging for young people to resist. Marketing through immersive environments is often purposely aimed at circumventing conscious processing of product attributes and eliciting emotional responses. Digital marketing routinely relies on implicit persuasion, involving mental processes, according to Nairn and Fine, that "are activated automatically and effortlessly, without intention or awareness, and are thus difficult to control."[84] If brands are embedded in an entertainment context, as with in-game advertising or other immersive environments, they can still be influential without being consciously recognized or recalled.[85–87]

Based on the industry's own research, these techniques can be highly successful in triggering positive online responses to advertising messages and increasing sales of brands marketed in immersive environments.[88,89] The McDonald's *Avatar* campaign is a prime example of such a successful strategy. It extended the brand experience—for both the film and the fast-food company—into an immersive online virtual environment that was its own interactive version of the movie, specially designed to engage children and teens for long periods of time and to associate the food products with the pleasure of the immersive experience. The company saw an 18% increase in US Big Mac sales as a result of the campaign, whose combined innovative digital elements, according to an award it received from a marketing industry trade association, generated "awareness, purchases, engagement [and] repeat visits."[2]

HEALTH IMPLICATIONS AND POLICY REMEDIES

Taken together—and viewed against the backdrop of the major changes occurring in the worlds of media, advertising, and market research—the several developments discussed in this article constitute a new direction that is fundamentally different from the ways in which advertising and marketing were conducted in the past. Because marketing to children is already a well-established, profitable industry, its imperatives are influencing the design of digital content and services for children and teens in fundamental ways.

There is sufficient evidence in the current scientific literature on child development and on children's responses to advertising to raise serious questions about many of the contemporary techniques marketers are using to target young people online.[90–92] Digital marketing routinely blurs the lines between content and advertising, making it more difficult for children to discern the commercial content in online environments.[92–94] Children's attention online "may be largely engaged with the interactive experience," explains child development scholar Louis Moses. As a consequence, their ability to attend consciously to the marketing techniques "may be processed only peripherally, and thereby less deeply."[91]

Even in cases when children recognize that marketers are trying to influence them, they may be thwarted in their understanding because of the powerful nature of digital marketing environments, which, according to Moses, are often "interactive, immersive, alluring, engaging, and motivationally and emotionally rewarding."[91] Despite the expansion in digital youth marketing, however, only a few scholarly studies have examined its impact on young people.[15,57,67,86,95–101]

A comprehensive research and policy agenda is needed to adequately address the growing digital marketplace. Intervention strategies need to be inclusive and multifaceted, involving a wide range of government, public health, advocacy, and industry stakeholders at state and federal levels. They need to take into account the full spectrum of advertising and marketing practices across all media. Through a combination of policy and self-regulatory activities, it may be possible to develop safeguards that address concerns raised by these new forms of digital marketing.

The Children's Online Privacy Protection Act (COPPA) provides a useful policy framework that may be adapted to cover some of the digital techniques used by food marketers to target young people. COPPA limits online marketers from collecting personal information from children under age 13.[102,103] The Federal Trade Commission is currently revising its COPPA regulations to address several of the changes in digital marketing described in this article. The commission's proposed changes could make it more difficult for advertisers to establish a one-to-one connection with children across a variety of new platforms, including mobile phones and interactive games, and could provide additional protections against some of the emerging data collection and marketing practices.[104]

Although industry self-regulatory programs have made some efforts to cover digital marketing, they have not addressed adequately the full spectrum of contemporary practices used to promote products to children and adolescents through digital media. For example, the National Advertising Review Council's Children's Advertising Review Unit, which has been in place since the 1970s, has guidelines that cover all advertising and marketing directed at children ages 12 and under. Except for the provisions required by federal law pertaining to online children's privacy, the guidelines include only a handful of minimal safeguards for digital marketing, and they have not been sufficiently updated to address the range of marketing applications routinely used on social networks, mobile phones, and other popular digital platforms.[105,106]

Researchers, policymakers, and health professionals need to focus particular attention on adolescents and children of color. The teen years are a critical developmental period, during which consumer and health behaviors are established that may last throughout an individual's life.[107,108] Although US advertising policy has a long tradition of regulatory and self-regulatory safeguards for children under age 12, teens have been largely overlooked in the regulatory arena.[109] A growing body of research, however, suggests that biologic and psychosocial attributes of adolescence may play an important role in how teens respond to marketing, making this age group more vulnerable than thought in the past.[110–112] African Americans and Hispanics are more engaged than whites in many new media platforms, a trend that is helping to fuel the growth of a large infrastructure of multicultural digital marketing designed to reach and engage this important demographic sector.[113–117] Marketing that is targeted at African American and Hispanic youth can have a particularly powerful impact on their consumption choices, health behaviors, and social norms.[118,119]

At the core of the new framework to protect children online should be a set of fair marketing principles and practices. They should be focused on all digital marketing targeted at both young children and adolescents. The goal should be to balance the ability of young people to participate fully in the digital media culture — as producers, consumers, and citizens — with the governmental and industry obligation to ensure that youth are not subjected to unfair and deceptive marketing, particularly for unhealthy products.

REFERENCES

1. McDonald's orders up augmented reality from total immersion in global promotion for Fox's Avatar. 2009. Available at: http://seriousgamesmarket.blogspot.com/2009/12/serious-games-as-ar-extensive.html. Accessed April 10, 2010.
2. 2010 REGGIE awards: McDonald's avatar program. Promotion Marketing Association; 2010. Available at: http://www.omnicontests3.com/pma_reggie_awards/omnigallery/entry/gallery_item_info.cfm?child=1&client_id=1&entry_id=312&competition_id=1&entrant_id=97&gallery_item_id=135. Accessed August 5, 2010.
3. Avatar at McDonald's: experience the thrill! McDonald's; 2009. Available at: http://www.aboutmcdonalds.com/mcd/stories/our_business/mcd_avatar.html. Accessed August 4, 2010.
4. McDonald's Big Mac joins Fox's 'AVATAR' to thrill fans nationwide. 2009. Available at: http://www.prnewswire.com/news-releases/mcdonaldsr-big-macr-joins-foxs-avatar-to-thrill-fans-nationwide-78680402.html. Accessed August 4, 2010.
5. Class action lawsuit targets McDonald's use of toys to market to children. 2010. Available at: http://www.cspinet.org/new/201012151.html. Accessed February 24, 2011.
6. Montgomery K. Safeguards for youth in the digital marketing ecosystem. In: Singer DG, Singer JL, editors. Handbook of children and the media. Thousand Oaks (CA): Sage Publications; 2011. p. 631–48.
7. MTVN Digital. Fans: teens. n.d. Available at: http://mtvndigital.com/fans/teens/teens.php. Accessed February 6, 2012.
8. Swallow E. Mattel launches digital campaign aiming to reunite Barbie & Ken. 2011. Available at: http://mashable.com/2011/02/04/reunite-barbie-ken/. Accessed February 6, 2012.
9. Rideout VJ, Foehr UG, Roberts DF. Generation M2: media in the lives of 8-18-year-olds. Kaiser Family Foundation Study. 2010. Available at: http://www.kff.org/entmedia/upload/8010.pdf. Accessed September 4, 2010.
10. Engagement: definitions and anatomy. Advertising Research Foundation; 2006. Available at: http://my.thearf.org/source/Orders/index.cfm?section=unknown&task=3&CATEGORY=PUB&PRODUCT_TYPE=SALES&SKU=PUB_ENGDA_E&DESCRIPTION=Publications&FindSpec=&CFTOKEN=73112952&continue=1&SEARCH_TYPE=find&StartRow=1&PageNum=1. Accessed October 2, 2008.

11. Advertising Research Foundation. Defining engagement initiative. n.d. Available at: http://www.thearf.org/assets/research-arf-initiatives-defining-engagement. Accessed October 2, 2008.

12. MI4 engagement validation research agenda. Advertising Research Foundation Council on Experiential Marketing; 2006. Available at: http://www.thearf.org/downloads/councils/experiential/2006-05-18_ARF_EXP_diforio.pdf. Accessed March 27, 2007.

13. Heath R. How do we predict advertising attention and engagement? 2007. Available at: https://www.bath.ac.uk/opus/bitstream/10247/286/1/2007-09.pdf. Accessed March 4, 2008.

14. Chester J, Cheyne A, Dorfman L. Peeking behind the curtain: food and marketing industry research supporting digital media marketing to children and adolescents. 2011. Available at: http://digitalads.org/documents/CDD_BMSG_Industry_Research.pdf. Accessed September 13, 2011.

15. Montgomery K, Grier S, Chester J, et al. Food marketing in the digital age: a conceptual framework and agenda for research. 2011. Available at: http://digitalads.org/documents/Digital_Food_Mktg_Conceptual_Model%20Report.pdf. Accessed January 25, 2012.

16. Jacobson M, Mazur LA. Marketing madness: a survival guide for a consumer society. Boulder (CO): Westview Press; 1995.

17. Linn S. Consuming kids: the hostile takeover of childhood. New York: New Press; 2004.

18. Schor JB. Born to buy: the commercialized child and the new consumer culture. New York: Scribner; 2004.

19. Montgomery K. Generation digital: politics, commerce and childhood in the age of the internet. Cambridge (MA): MIT Press; 2007.

20. Advertising Research Foundation. Council on youth advertising. n.d. Available at: http://www.thearf.org/assets/youth-council. Accessed March 27, 2007.

21. Truly, madly, deeply engaged: global youth, media and technology. Yahoo & OMD; 2005. Available at: http://us.yimg.com/i/adv/tmde_05/truly_madly_final_booklet.pdf. Accessed March 27, 2007.

22. Lippe D. It's all in creative delivery: gurus in the teen universe build a track record by gauging where the market is going. Advert Age 2001;26:S8–9.

23. Chester J, Montgomery K. Interactive food & beverage marketing: targeting children and youth in the digital age. 2007. Available at: http://www.digitalads.org/documents/digiMarketingFull.pdf. Accessed May 19, 2010.

24. Chester J, Montgomery K. Interactive food & beverage marketing: targeting children and youth in the digital age: an update. 2008. Available at: http://digitalads.org/documents/NPLAN_digital_mktg_memo.pdf. Accessed January 21, 2012.

25. Yahoo. Yahoo! Messenger—imvironments: food and drink. n.d. Available at: http://messenger.yahoo.com/imv.php;_ylt=AhP4H.Kjy3g_DYV38XSyiIRqMMIF?cat=Food%20and%20Drink. Accessed October 2, 2008.

26. Crupi A. Upfront: the kids are all right: younger set's bizarre expected to top $1 billion. Adweek; 2011. Available at: http://www.adweek.com/news/advertising-branding/upfront-kids-are-all-right-126382. Accessed October 2, 2011.

27. Braiker B. The next great American consumer: infants to 3-year-olds: they're a new demographic marketers are hell-bent on reaching. Adweek; 2011. Available at: http://www.adweek.com/news/advertising-branding/next-great-american-consumer-135207. Accessed October 2, 2011.

28. US child social network users, by age. eMarketer; 2011. Available at: http://www.emarketer.com/Products/Explore/Search.aspx?dsNav=Rpp:25. Nrc:id-1048, N:701–718. Accessed January 25, 2012.

29. Neff J. Cybertots: pre-teens drive iPad purchases, join social networks. Advert Age 2011. Available at: http://adage.com/article/news/pre-teens-drive-ipad-purchases-join-social-networks/227101/. Accessed October 2, 2011.

30. Lenhart A, Purcell K, Smith A, et al. Social media and young adults. 2010. Available at: http://www.pewinternet.org/Reports/2010/Social-Media-and-Young-Adults.aspx. Accessed March 23, 2011.

31. Owyang J. A collection of social network stats for 2010. Available at: http://www.web-strategist.com/blog/2010/01/19/a-collection-of-social-network-stats-for-2010/. Accessed March 13, 2010.

32. Marcus H, Nurius P. Possible selves. Am Psychol 1986;41:954–69.

33. Stern S. Producing sites: exploring identities: youth online authorship. In: Buckingham D, editor. Youth, identity, and digital media. Cambridge (MA): MIT Press; 2007. p. 99–117.

34. Buckingham D, editor. Youth, identity, and digital media. Cambridge (MA): MIT Press; 2007.

35. IAB platform status report: user generated content, social media, and advertising—an overview. Interactive Advertising Bureau; 2008. Available at: http://www.iab.net/media/file/2008_ugc_platform.pdf. Accessed September 12, 2010.

36. Social media metrics definitions. Interactive Advertising Bureau; 2009. Available at: http://www.slideshare.net/womarketing/iab-social-media-metrics-definitions. Accessed September 13, 2011.

37. Social media buyer's guide. Interactive Advertising Bureau; 2010. Available at: http://www.iab.net/media/file/IAB_SocialMedia_Booklet.pdf. Accessed September 13, 2011.

38. Iskold A. Social graph: concepts and issues. Readwriteweb; 2007. Available at: http://www.readwriteweb.com/archives/social_graph_concepts_and_issues.php. Accessed October 2, 2008.

39. Montgomery K, Chester J. Digital food marketing to children and youth: problematic practices and policy interventions. 2011. Available at: http://case-studies.digitalads.org/wp-content/uploads/2011/10/DigitalMarketingReport_FINAL_web_20111017.pdf. Accessed January 25, 2012.

40. Global social network advertising market to reach US$14.8 billion by 2017, according to a new report by Global Industry Analysts, Inc. 2011. Available at: http://www.digitaljournal.com/pr/446579. Accessed October 27, 2011.

41. Yap J. Social media revenue to hit US$29b by 2015. Zdnet; 2011. Available at: http://www.zdnetasia.com/social-media-revenue-to-hit-us29b-by-2015-62302471.htm. Accessed Oct. 27, 2011.

42. Kaplan D. Magna: online, TV ad gains hold steady as wider recovery slows. 2011. Available at: http://paidcontent.org/article/419-magna-online-tv-ad-gains-hold-steady-as-wider-recovery-slows-/. Accessed October 27, 2011.

43. Hardawar D. Google acquires Invite Media to help users with ad exchanges. Venturebeat; 2010. Available at: http://venturebeat.com/2010/06/02/google-acquires-invite-media-to-help-users-with-ad-exchanges/. Accessed February 15, 2011.

44. Kaplan D. VC money keeps pouring in for ad targeters: turn raises $20 million. 2011. Available at: http://paidcontent.org/article/419-vc-money-keeps-pouring-in-for-ad-targeters-turn-raises-20-million/. Accessed February 15, 2011.

45. Demand-side platforms buyer's guide. Econsultancy; 2011. Available at: http://econsultancy.com/us/reports/dsps-buyers-guide. Accessed September 13, 2011.

46. Center for Digital Democracy, U.S. PIRG, World Privacy Forum. In the matter of real-time targeting and auctioning, data profiling optimization, and economic loss to consumers and privacy, complaint, request for investigation, injunction,

and other relief: Google, Yahoo, Pubmatic, Targusinfo, Mediamath, Exelate, Rubicon Project, Appnexus, Rocket Fuel, and others named below. Federal Trade Commission filing. 2010. Available at: http://www.democraticmedia.org/real-time-targeting. Accessed February 9, 2011.

47. Butterfinger—Comedy Network. n.d. Available at: http://comedy.video.yahoo.com/. Accessed September 13, 2011.

48. Stecklow S. On the web, children face intensive tracking. Wall St J 2010. Available at: http://online.wsj.com/article/SB10001424052748703904304575497903523187146.html. Accessed September 17, 2011.

49. Hof RD. Ad networks are transforming online advertising. BusinessWeek; 2009. Available at: http://www.businessweek.com/magazine/content/09_09/b4121048726676.htm. Accessed October 2, 2011.

50. New research reveals widespread tracking and behavioral targeting on children's websites; groups call on FTC to update online privacy safeguards for children. Center for Digital Democracy; 2011. Available at: http://www.democraticmedia.org/new-research-reveals-widespread-tracking-and-behavioral-targeting-children's-websites-groups-call-ft. Accessed February 6, 2012.

51. Bell J. Brands: claim your Facebook place today. 2010. Available at: http://johnbell.typepad.com/weblog/2010/08/brands-claim-your-facebook-place-today.html. Accessed December 31, 2010.

52. Hansen EJ. How to optimize mobile marketing efforts with targeting. 2010. Available at: http://www.mobilemarketer.com/cms/opinion/columns/8347.html. Accessed January 3, 2011.

53. Vdopia. n.d. Available at: http://www.ivdopia.com/?page=insights. Accessed January 3, 2011.

54. comScore reports July 2011 U.S. mobile subscriber market share. Available at: http://www.comscore.com/Press_Events/Press_Releases/2011/8/comScore_Reports_July_2011_U.S._Mobile_Subscriber_Market_Share. Accessed September 13, 2011.

55. Kellogg D. 40 percent of U.S. mobile users own smartphones; 40 percent are Android. 2011. Available at: http://blog.nielsen.com/nielsenwire/?p=28790. Accessed September 13, 2011.

56. Christian L, Keeter S, Purcell K, et al. Assessing the cell phone challenge. 2010. Available at: http://pewresearch.org/pubs/1601/assessing-cell-phone-challenge-in-public-opinion-surveys. Accessed February 23, 2011.

57. Daily media use among children and teens up dramatically from five years ago. Kaiser Family Foundation; 2010. Available at: http://www.kff.org/entmedia/entmedia012010nr.cfm. Accessed April 7, 2010.

58. eMarketer. Mobile phone activities of US children, 2009 & 2011. Available at: http://www.emarketer.com/Products/Explore/Search.aspx?dsNav=Rpp:25, Nrc:id-1048, N:718-851. Accessed January 25, 2011.

59. U.S. parents say almost a third of the apps on their phone were downloaded by their children. 2011. Available at: http://blog.nielsen.com/nielsenwire/online_mobile/u-s-parents-say-almost-a-third-of-the-apps-on-their-phone-were-downloaded-their-children/. Accessed October 2, 2011.

60. Interactive food & beverage marketing: targeting children and youth in the digital age. n.d. Available at: http://www.digitalads.org/findrecords.php. Accessed October 2, 2011.

61. Gutnick AL, Robb M, Takeuchi L, et al. Always connected: the new digital media habits of young children. 2011. Available at: http://joanganzcooneycenter.org/Reports-28.html. Accessed January 25, 2012.

62. Pearson-McNeil C, Hale T. Dissecting diversity: understanding the ethnic consumer. 2011. Available at: http://blog.nielsen.com/nielsenwire/consumer/dissecting-diversity-understanding-the-ethnic-consumer/print/. Accessed October 2, 2011.

63. More Americans watching mobile video. Nielsen Company; 2010. Available at: http://blog.nielsen.com/nielsenwire/online_mobile/americans-watch-more-mobile-video-now-than-ever/. Accessed December 31, 2010.

64. U.S. teen mobile report: calling yesterday, texting today, using apps tomorrow. Nielsen Company; 2010. Available at: http://blog.nielsen.com/nielsenwire/online_mobile/u-s-teen-mobile-report-calling-yesterday-texting-today-using-apps-tomorrow/. Accessed January 3, 2011.

65. MMA mobile advertising guidelines. Mobile Marketing Association; 2011. Available at: http://www.mmaglobal.com/mobilecouponguidelines.pdf. Accessed September 14, 2011.

66. Apsalar. Aptimizer. n.d. Available at: http://apsalar.com/documentation/aptimizer/. Accessed September 14, 2011.

67. Rao L. Google sites now allows you to create a mobile landing page. TechCrunch; 2011. Available at: http://techcrunch.com/2011/06/29/google-sites-now-allows-you-to-create-a-mobile-landing-page/. Accessed September 14, 2011.

68. mobiThinking. Global mobile statistics 2012: all quality mobile marketing research, mobile web stats, subscribers, ad revenue, usage, trends.... Available at: http://mobithinking.com/mobile-marketing-tools/latest-mobile-stats#lotsofapps. Accessed January 25, 2012.

69. Patel K. Fast-food chains grab most location-based check-ins. Advert Age 2010. Available at: http://adage.com/digital/article?article_id=145413. Accessed January 3, 2011.

70. The mobile path to purchase. DDB; 2011. Available at: http://www.ddb.com/ddblogs/strategy/the-mobile-path-to-purchase.html. Accessed September 14, 2011.

71. Thomson J. Internet and interactive games tipped to drive media sector growth. SmartCompany; 2010. Available at: http://www.smartcompany.com.au/media/20100802-internet-and-interactive-games-tipped-to-drive-media-sector-growth.html. Accessed August 26, 2010.

72. Ogden G. Study: online game revenue to fuel market growth. Edge Magazine; 2010. Available at: http://www.edge-online.com/news/study-online-game-revenue-to-fuel-market-growth. Accessed August 26, 2010.

73. Parfitt B. 360 claims half of all online console gaming. MCV; 2009. Available at: http://www.mcvuk.com/news/33490/360-claims-half-of-all-online-console-gaming. Accessed August 26, 2010.

74. Varney A. Immersion unexplained. The Escapist; 2006. Available at: http://www.escapistmagazine.com/articles/view/issues/issue_57/341-Immersion-Unexplained. Accessed August 26, 2010.

75. Cowley B, Charles D, Black M, et al. Toward an understanding of flow in video games. Comput Entertain 2008;6:1–27.

76. Gaudiosi J. Google gets in-game with adscape. The Hollywood Reporter; 2007. Available at: http://www.hollywoodreporter.com/hr/content_display/business/news/e3i898ca0de1754206ae43bdbc6ee2d9ffd. Accessed October 2, 2008.

77. Shields M. In-game ads could reach $2 bil. Adweek; 2006. Available at: http://www.adweek.com/aw/national/article_display.jsp?vnu_content_id=1002343563. Accessed October 2, 2008.

78. Dickson D. New research study: advertising engagement in digital magazines. 2011. Available at: http://blogs.adobe.com/digitalpublishing/2011/01/ad-engagement.html. Accessed September 13, 2011.

79. Hoffman DL, Novak TP. Marketing in hypermedia computer-mediated environments: conceptual foundations. J Market 1996;60:50–68.

80. Wang A. Digital ad engagement: perceived interactivity as a driver of advertising effectiveness. 2011. Available at: http://blogs.adobe.com/digitalpublishing/files/2011/01/digital_magazine_ad_engagement.pdf. Accessed September 13, 2011.

81. Advertising Age. Ad networks + exchanges guide. 2010. Available at: http://brandedcontent.adage.com/adnetworkguide10/. Accessed September 13, 2011.

82. Dart Motif. Sites—overview. n.d. Available at: http://www.dartmotif.com/sites/sites.asp. Accessed March 30, 2007.

83. MC insight: advertising and video games. Havas Digital; 2008. Available at: http://www.mediacontacts.com/2008/07/advertising-and-video-games/. Accessed September 13, 2011.

84. Nairn A, Fine C. Who's messing with my mind? The implications of dual-process models for the ethics of advertising to children. Int J Advert 2008;27:447–70.

85. Auty S, Lewis C. The 'delicious paradox': preconscious processing of product placements by children. In: Shrum LJ, editor. The psychology of entertainment media: blurring the lines between entertainment and persuasion. London: Psychology Press; 2003. p. 117–33.

86. Harris JL, Brownell KD, Bargh JA. The food marketing defense model: integrating psychological research to protect youth and inform public policy. Soc Issues Policy Rev 2009;3:211–71.

87. Law S, Braun KA. I'll have what she's having: gauging the impact of product placements on viewers. Psychol Market 2000;17:1059–75.

88. Kroese M. Is it what you watch... or who you are?—IAB Mixx 2010. Available at: http://community.microsoftadvertising.com/blogs/advertising/archive/2010/09/10/is-it-what-you-watch-or-who-you-are.aspx. Accessed February 22, 2011.

89. Microsoft Advertising. Xbox. n.d. Available at: http://advertising.microsoft.com/gaming/xbox-advertising. Accessed September 13, 2011.

90. Cai X, Zhao X. Click here, kids! Online advertising practices on popular children's websites. J Child Media 2010;4:135–54.

91. Moses LJ. Research on child development: implications for how children understand and cope with digital media. Memo prepared for the second NPLAN/BMSG meeting on digital media and marketing to children for the NPLAN marketing to children learning community. 2009. Available at: http://www.digitalads.org/documents/Moses_NPLAN_BMSG_memo.pdf. Accessed February 22, 2011.

92. Kunkel D, Castonguay J. Children and advertising: content, comprehension, and consequences. In: Singer DG, Singer JL, editors. Handbook of children and the media. Thousand Oaks (CA): Sage Publications; 2012. p.

93. Ali M, Blades M, Oates MC, et al. Young children's ability to recognize advertisements in web page designs. Br J Dev Psychol 2009;27:71–83.

94. McIlrath M. Children's cognitive processing of Internet advertising [PhD dissertation, University of California at Santa Barbara, Department of Communication]. 2006.

95. Alvy LM, Calvert SL. Food marketing on popular children's web sites: a content analysis. J Am Diet Assoc 2008;108:710–3.

96. American Academy of Pediatrics Committee on Communications. Policy statement: children, adolescents, and advertising. Pediatrics 2006;118:2563–9.

97. Calvert SL. Children as consumers: advertising and marketing. Future Child 2008;18:205–34.

98. Calvert SL, Jordan AB, Cocking RR, editors. Children in the digital age: influences of electronic media on development. Westport (CT): Praeger; 2002.

99. Kunkel D, Wilcox BL, Cantor J, et al. Report of the APA task force on advertising and children. 2004. Available at: http://www.kff.org/entmedia/upload/The-Role-Of-Media-in-Childhood-Obesity.pdf. Accessed October 2, 2008.

100. Moore ES. It's child's play: advergaming and the online marketing of food to children. 2006. Available at: http://www.kff.org/entmedia/upload/7536.pdf. Accessed October 2, 2008.

101. Moore ES, Rideout VJ. The online marketing of food to children: is it just fun and games? J Publ Pol Market 2007;6:202–20.

102. Miyazaki AD, Stanaland AJ, Lwin MO. Self-regulatory safeguards and the online privacy of preteen children. J Advert 2009;38:79–83.

103. Stanaland AJS, Lwin MO, Leong S. Providing parents with online privacy information: approaches in the US and the UK. J Consum Aff 2009;42(3):474, 484–5.

104. FTC seeks comment on proposed revisions to children's online privacy protection rule. Federal Trade Commission; 2011. Available at: http://www.ftc.gov/opa/2011/09/coppa.shtm. Accessed February 6, 2012.

105. Self-regulatory program for children's advertising. Children's Advertising Review Unit; 2006. Available at: http://www.caru.org/guidelines/guidelines.pdf. Accessed February 26, 2011.

106. Kelley B. Industry controls over food marketing to children: are they effective? Public Health Advocacy Institute; 2005. Available at: http://www.aeforum.org/aeforum.nsf/88e10e9813be5a4780256c5100355eb1/75633673317e30f28025704300350d77/$FILE/PHAI.caru.analysis.pdf. Accessed February 26, 2011.

107. Brownell KD, Schwartz MB, Puhl RM, et al. The need for bold action to prevent adolescent obesity. J Adolesc Health 2009;45:S8–17.

108. Story M, Sallis J, Orleans T. Adolescent obesity: toward evidence-based policy and environmental solutions. J Adolesc Health 2009;45:S1–5.

109. Matecki LA. Update: COPPA is ineffective legislation! Next steps for protecting youth privacy rights in the social networking era. Northwest J Law Soc Pol 2010; 5:369–402.

110. Leslie FM, Levine LJ, Loughlin SE, et al. Adolescents' psychological & neurobiological development: Implications for digital marketing. Memo prepared for the second NPLAN/BMSG meeting on digital media and marketing to children for the NPLAN marketing to children learning community. 2009. Available at: http://digitalads.org/documents/Leslie_et_al_NPLAN_BMSG_memo.pdf. Accessed August 26, 2010.

111. Montgomery K, Chester J. Interactive food & beverage marketing: targeting adolescents in the digital age. J Adolesc Health 2009;45:S18–29.

112. Pechmann C, Levine L, Loughlin S, et al. Impulsive and self-conscious: adolescents' vulnerability to advertising and promotion. J Publ Pol Market 2005;24: 202–21.

113. Billingsley LG. Social media is the new avenue to reach multicultural audiences. PRWeek; 2009. Available at: http://www.prweekus.com/pages/Login.aspx?retUrl=/Social-media-is-the-new-avenue-to-reach-multicultural-audiences/article/131349/&PageTypeId=28&ArticleId=131349&accessLevel=2. Accessed February 27, 2011.

114. Lopez MH, Livingston G. How young Latinos communicate with friends in the digital age. Pew Hispanic Center; 2010. Available at: http://pewhispanic.org/files/reports/124.pdf. Accessed February 27, 2011.

115. Black America today: the future, the past, the present. Radio One; 2008. Available at: http://blackamericastudy.com/summary/AA-Presentation-Public-Deck-3.pd. Accessed February 6, 2012.

116. Smith A. Who's on what: social media trends among communities of color. Pew Internet & American Life Project; 2011. Available at: http://www.pewinternet.org/Presentations/2011/Jan/Social-Media-Trends-Among-Communities-of-Color.aspx. Accessed February 6, 2012.
117. Villa J. 2011: the year of creative destruction. Engage: Hispanics. 2011. Available at: http://www.mediapost.com/publications/index.cfm?fa=Articles.showArticle&art_aid=142461. Accessed February 6, 2012.
118. Grier SA, Mensinger J, et al. Fast food marketing and children's fast food consumption: exploring parental influences in an ethnically diverse sample. J Publ Pol Market 2007;26:221–35.
119. Grier S, Kumanyika S. The context for choice: health implications of targeted food and beverage marketing to African Americans. Am J Public Health 2008;98:1616–29.

Childhood Obesity and the Media

Melanie Hingle, PhD, MPH, RD[a],*, Dale Kunkel, PhD[b]

KEYWORDS

- Childhood obesity • Media • Communication • Food advertising • Policy

KEY POINTS

- Electronic media use is significantly positively correlated with adiposity in children.
- Interventions reducing screen media use by children (eg, eliminating television from children's bedrooms; turning off the television while eating) have been associated with improvement in child weight status.
- Children's exposure to media marketing messages for unhealthy food products is well established as a significant contributor to childhood obesity.
- Food industry self-regulation initiatives have had only negligible effects in improving the nutritional quality of foods advertised to children.

An epidemic of childhood obesity afflicts American youth (**Fig. 1**). Approximately 32% of children and adolescents aged 2 to 19 years are overweight (body mass index [BMI] $\geq$85th percentile for children of the same age and sex), and 17% (or 12.5 million) of these children are considered obese (BMI $\geq$95th percentile for children of the same age and sex).[1] Adiposity poses risks for significant adverse health consequences. Obese children are more likely than normal-weight children to have hypertension and high cholesterol,[2] impaired glucose tolerance, insulin resistance, type 2 diabetes,[3] sleep apnea and asthma,[4,5] joint problems,[6] fatty liver, gallstones, gastroesophageal reflux,[3–5] as well as increased risk of social and psychological problems such as poor self-esteem and discrimination.[3,7,8] Obesity in childhood has been shown to track into adulthood, placing obese children at risk of future weight-related diseases.[9,10]

Numerous elements contribute to childhood obesity. Regular consumption of a calorie-dense, nutrient-poor diet and inadequate moderate-to-vigorous physical activity are key risk factors. Media use has also been established as a strong correlate of childhood obesity. This relationship was first identified in the 1980s[11] and has been

[a] Department of Nutritional Sciences, University of Arizona, 1177 East, 4th Street, Shantz Building, Room 328, Tucson, AZ 85721, USA; [b] Department of Communication, University of Arizona, 1103 East, University Boulevard, P.O. Box 210025, Tucson, AZ 85721, USA
* Corresponding author.
E-mail address: hinglem@email.arizona.edu

Pediatr Clin N Am 59 (2012) 677–692
doi:10.1016/j.pcl.2012.03.021
0031-3955/12/$ – see front matter © 2012 Elsevier Inc. All rights reserved.

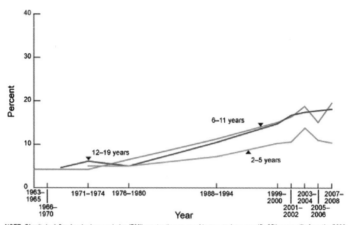

Fig. 1. Prevalence of obesity among children and adolescents, by age group, United States, 1963 to 2008. (*From* Ogden CL, Carroll M. Prevalence of obesity among children and adolescents: United States, trends 1963–1965 through 2007–2008. NCH Health E-Stats. CDC/National Center for Health Statistics; 2010. Available at http://www.cdc.gov/nchs/data/hestat/obesity_child_07_08/obesity_child_07_08.htm.)

corroborated by dozens of studies since then.[12,13] It is often assumed that the sedentary nature of television viewing, traditionally the largest component of young people's time spent with media, is the mechanism underlying the relationship. The presumption holds that heavy media users are transformed into so-called couch potatoes who devote insufficient time to exercise because their eyes are too often glued to the screen.[14,15] Consistent with this perspective, the US Department of Health and Human Services specified a national objective of reducing television viewing to combat obesity in its *Healthy People 2010* target goals.[16]

However, more recent evidence has focused increasing attention on the role of food marketing to children as a causal factor contributing to childhood obesity.[17] Given the significant amount of time children spend watching television, they inevitably encounter large amounts of commercials for food products.[18] Televised food advertising is dominated by high-density, low-nutrient products that the public typically labels as junk food.[19,20] Advertising for unhealthy food products has also migrated to new media venues frequented by children and teens, such as the Internet.[21–23] Exposure to commercial promotions in the media wields influence on children's food product preferences, requests, diet, and ultimately their diet-related health.[24] Advertising exposure may be the principal causal mechanism that explains why screen time is significantly correlated with childhood obesity, rather than the widely presumed couch-potato hypothesis.

This review article surveys the research that documents children's patterns of media use, analyzes the evidence that shows the association between young people's screen time and weight status, considers the role of food marketing as a contributor to childhood obesity, and evaluates recent intervention efforts intended to reduce children's screen time and/or exposure to advertising messages for unhealthy food products. Overall conclusions and possible solutions to reduce the role of media as a contributor to childhood obesity are also discussed.

SCREEN TIME WITHIN THE CONTEXT OF OBESITY PREVENTION

Screen time is a term meant to represent an individual's use of electronic mass media, including television viewing, video and computer game playing, DVD viewing, Internet use, and other online activities. Media use in childhood is primarily a means of entertainment, and hence is engaged in mostly during unstructured time outside of school hours.[25] Public health researchers originally conceived of screen time as a sedentary activity, which holds obvious implications for displacing time that might otherwise be devoted to physical exercise.

Given the recent proliferation of mobile technologies and digital media, screen time can now occur from almost any geographic location via highly portable video-enabled and Internet-enabled devices such as iPads, iPods, and smartphones. The use of these mobile technologies reduces the likelihood that the user is necessarily sedentary while engaging in screen-related activities, thus rendering the construct of screen time a less precise and reliable assessment of time spent in sedentary pursuits. However, regardless of how screen time may be defined and quantified, there is little doubt that children and adolescents spend significant time with screen-based media, and that media use by youth has increased as mobile technologies have become more readily available and accessible.[26]

Screen Media Diet: Infants and Preschoolers

Survey data indicate that television viewing begins at a young age,[27] and has surged as a function of the recent expansion in programming targeted specifically at infants.[28] More than half (59%) of children less than 2 years of age watch television on an average day,[29] despite the American Academy of Pediatrics recommending no media exposure before the age of 2 years.[30] Children average 2.2 hours of viewing per day at age 1 year, increasing to 3.6 hours per day by 3 years of age.[31] By age 5 years, more than 60% have used handheld games, 81% have played console games, and 90% have used a computer.[32]

Among children less than 8 years of age, most screen time is still spent watching television (74% of media time), followed by the use of computers (13%), video games (10% of the time), and , cell phones/iPods/iPads (4%).[32] Nearly half (47%) of children aged 5 to 8 years have a television set in their bedroom, including 30% of children less than 2 years old. Overall, the average daily time that children less than 8 years old spend with television and DVDs is estimated to be about 1:40, with roughly another half hour devoted to playing video, computer, or handheld games.[16,32]

Screen Media Diet: School-aged Children and Teens

The amount of time spent with media is also increasing for older children and adolescents. From 2005 to 2010, media use for those aged 8 to 18 years increased by more than an hour a day, moving from 6:21 to 7:38 daily.[25] As with younger children, most screen time was devoted to television. Older children and teens are more likely to multitask, in terms of engaging multiple media venues simultaneously, as well as engaging in activities such as homework while also using mass media.[33] Older children and teens spend more time with media than in any other waking activity. As Rideout and colleagues[25] observed, using media comprises a full-time job for youth, accounting for 7.5 hours per day, 7 days per week.

Although there may be some benefits associated with children's screen media use, such as learning from educational programs, there is also significant risk for a range of adverse side effects. Exposure to certain types of media portrayals may increase child viewers' aggressive behavior,[34] decrease the age of first sexual intercourse,[35] and contribute to gender[36] and ethnic group stereotyping[37] in children and teens. However, regardless of the type of content viewed, heavy screen media use correlates significantly with overweight and obesity in children.

ASSOCIATION BETWEEN SCREEN TIME AND OBESITY IN CHILDREN AND ADOLESCENTS

A systematic review of the published research evidence linking television exposure with adiposity was conducted in 2006 by the Institute of Medicine (IOM).[24] The IOM identified more than 60 studies conducted over roughly the past 20 years that converged to show a small but statistically significant relationship between television exposure and child obesity. Studies were evaluated for methodological strength, and the greater the study's rigor, the greater the likelihood that it showed a significant relationship between these variables. Since the IOM review was published, numerous large-scale epidemiologic studies have emerged to further corroborate this relationship.[38–42]

Data from cross-sectional and longitudinal studies yield the same pattern of results. One review of research reported that, in 18 of 22 longitudinal studies, more hours of media exposure predicted increased weight over time.[43] Although a small minority of studies have produced nonsignificant results, the null findings are most often attributed to limitations in defining and measuring time spent with screen media,[26,44] among other confounds. One of these complications involves video game use.

Video Games

By most definitions, screen time encompasses video game play. However, studies that focused on video game play have been less consistent in showing correlations between screen time and adiposity, compared with research centered on television use.[16] Fewer studies have specifically targeted video game play, and, although some of these yield evidence of associations with obesity,[45,46] others do not.[47,48] A recent review of evidence found that there were more studies that produced no significant association between video game play and obesity than had yielded significant correlations.[49] One of the most obvious complications here is that video games are not as inherently sedentary as watching television,[50,51] especially when exercise-oriented games such as *Dance Dance Revolution* are considered.[52]

Possible Causal Mechanisms

The direction of causality in the relationship between screen time and obesity could potentially flow either way. That is, overweight individuals might tend to stay home and use media more than physically active people, hence accounting for the relationship between screen time and adiposity. Although plausible, this possibility is rebutted by several types of evidence. Twelve of 15 longitudinal studies that measure television use at time 1 and weight status at 1 or more subsequent points in time produced significant associations with weight gain over time.[24] In addition, an experimental intervention that reduced screen time over a 6-month period found significantly less increase in BMI and other measures of adiposity, compared with a control group.[53] The totality of evidence suggests that greater amounts of time spent with screen media lead to weight gain and the risk of obesity, rather than the other way around. What is less clear is the underlying mechanism that accounts for that relationship.

Data that merely correlate media use with childhood obesity do not clarify whether weight gain may be a function of the largely sedentary nature of the activity (ie, displacement of physically active time), or might instead be the result of some other factor/s. There are several incongruities that pose challenges for the couch-potato hypothesis. The American Academy of Pediatrics[54] has observed that, although many studies find that physical activity decreases as screen time increases,[39,55,56] many others do not.[57–59] Within child care settings, for example, 1 study found that youngsters attending day care centers with high use of electronic media had greater sedentary behavior than children in centers with low electronic media use,[60] but 2 other comparable studies found no association between these variables.[61,62]

Higher levels of screen time do not always correlate with lower levels of physical activity. An IOM review reported only 14 of 20 studies that analyzed these variables found a significant relationship (see Table 5-22 in Ref.[24]). It is common for studies to find only small proportions of children that concomitantly experience high screen time and low physical activity. For example, in one study of children aged 4 to 11 years using National Health and Nutrition Examination Survey (NHANES) data (N = 2964), less than one-quarter of boys (23.7%) and one-third of girls (29.1%) were in this category.[63] In addition, most studies that control statistically for amount of physical activity in examining the relationship between screen time and obesity still produce a significant correlation.

Perhaps the most telling evidence is provided by a study that separated time spent watching television into 2 categories, 1 with and 1 without commercial advertisements included.[42] The findings were clear. Time spent viewing commercial television was significantly correlated with BMI, whereas time watching noncommercial television was not. The overall evidence in this area clearly suggests that the role of media in contributing to childhood obesity entails more than simply displacing time that would otherwise be devoted to exercise. Another factor that may play a role involves snacking that occurs during television viewing time. However, the most likely alternative explanation for the linkage between screen time and adiposity involves the influence of advertisements for unhealthy foods that are widespread in media consumed by children.

THE ROLE OF FOOD MARKETING IN CHILDHOOD OBESITY

As indicated earlier, children engage in heavy media use, with television still dominant among an increasingly diverse range of screen media. Given that commercial messages are pervasive in most television content, it is inevitable that child viewers are exposed to large numbers of advertisements, including many for food products. According to the Federal Trade Commission, children aged 2 to 17 years see roughly 5500 televised food advertisements per year, or about 15.1 per day.[64] Commercials for food products have long been a staple in children's television programming, and the featured items are typically low-nutrient, calorie-dense fast foods, candies, snacks, and sugared cereals.[65,66]

Food Advertising to Children

Food marketers invest nearly $2 billion annually in child-targeted advertising, with the largest share devoted to television advertisements.[67] Studies of advertising content document the prevalence of obesogenic foods in television advertising targeted at youth.[66,68] For example, 2 out of every 3 cereals (66%) advertised to children fail to meet nutritional standards with regard to added sugar.[69] Nearly all (98%) food advertisements seen by children and 89% viewed by adolescents are for products high in fat, sugar, or sodium (**Fig. 2**).[19] In contrast, healthy foods that should be part of a regular diet are almost never advertised to children.[19,70,71]

As new media have evolved and attracted children's interest, advertisers have migrated to these venues along with youth audiences. Food marketers have

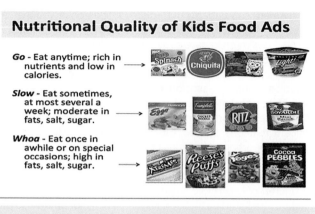

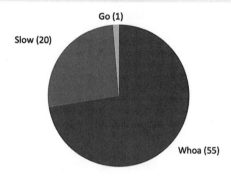

Nutritional Quality of Food Ads in 10 Hours of Children's Programming

Fig. 2. Nutritional quality of foods advertised in children's programming. (*From* Kunkel D, McKinley C, Wright P. Assessing compliance with industry self-regulation of televised food marketing to children. Oakland (CA): Children Now; 2009; with permission.)

established Internet Web sites that offer games and other attractive entertainment options for children, creating a media experience that is a commercial promotion.[21,72,73] Product-based so-called advergames allow children to play virtual games with popular brand characters such as Chester Cheeto or Tony the Tiger,[22] blurring boundaries between commercial and entertainment content in a manner that federal regulations prohibit on television.[74] More than half of the food advertisements on children's television programs now promote such product-based Web sites.[75]

Other innovations in marketing food products to children include in-game advertising, placed within video games[76]; viral marketing, in which consumers share product-related messages with friends to receive rewards[77]; and promotional activities in schools.[78] Collectively, these efforts comprise a significant expansion of the overall commercial environment targeted at youth, which many now describe as the commercialization of childhood.[79–81]

Effects of Food Advertising on Children

Food marketing plays a significant role in shaping children's nutritional knowledge, eating habits, and weight status. Heavy exposure to televised food advertising is associated with nutritional misperceptions: the greater the exposure to food advertising, the greater the likelihood that unhealthy items will be judged as healthy and nutritious.[82–84] Numerous experiments show short-term effects on children's attitudes and product preferences for foods.[18,85] Amount of television exposure is positively correlated with children's ability to correctly identify product brands[86] and with their consumption of advertised brands.[87]

The most comprehensive review of studies examining the effects of food marketing on children was conducted by the IOM in 2006. The IOM report concluded that (1) there is strong evidence that advertising influences the short-term food consumption of children aged 2 to 11 years; (2) there is moderate evidence that advertising influences the regular diet of children 2 to 5 years of age, and weak evidence (ie, more studies are needed) that it influences children 6 to 11 years of age; and (3) there is strong evidence that exposure to advertising is associated with adiposity in children 2 to 11 years of age and teens 12 to 18 years of age. The report summarized its findings by observing that "food and beverage marketing practices geared to children and youth are out of balance with healthful diets, and contribute to an environment that puts their health at risk."[24(p374)]

The conclusion that advertising to children works as intended is clear, if unremarkable.[18] In an ideal world, parents would refuse children's purchase influence requests for unhealthy foods, negating much of the impact of advertising. In practice, parents have a high rate of yielding to children's requests.[88,89] Furthermore, most children begin to purchase snack foods with their own money as early as 8 years of age.[90] Thus, given that children's exposure to media marketing messages for unhealthy food products is now well established as a significant contributor to childhood obesity, this article reviews possible tactics and strategies that might mitigate the health risks posed in this area.

REDUCING MEDIA CONTRIBUTIONS TO CHILDHOOD OBESITY

There are 2 distinct approaches to ameliorating the role that media play in contributing to childhood obesity. The first involves individual-level interventions that seek to reduce children's screen time. The second involves institutional-level efforts to diminish children's exposure to unhealthy food advertising by limiting its presence in young people's media environment. This article addresses each of these topics in turn.

Interventions to Limit Screen Time

Since Dietz and Gortmaker's[11] influential work describing the association between television viewing and childhood obesity, a large number of intervention programs have been conducted seeking to reduce children's screen time as a means to influence adiposity. Although some of these efforts have focused on screen time reduction, most have addressed media use within the context of a healthy lifestyle intervention that also included strategies to improve diet and physical activity. Given our focus on the role of media in childhood obesity, discussion of the intervention literature in this article is limited to media use issues only.

One of the first noteworthy experiments to focus on the effects of reducing screen time on obesity was conducted by Thomas Robinson[53] in the late 1990s. This randomized controlled trial consisted of a series of 18 lessons (30–50 minutes in length) taught by trained third and fourth grade classroom teachers over a period of 6 months, along with the use of an electronic device to assist participants in monitoring their media time. The intervention group achieved significant reductions in time devoted to media, an outcome that was linked to reductions in several measures of adiposity. The reduction in adiposity was achieved without any significant change in moderate-to-vigorous physical activity levels by the treatment group.

Subsequent studies have corroborated the finding that interventions that prove successful at reducing screen time typically achieve significant improvements in weight status.[91–95] Like the initial Robinson[53] trial, most observe that this outcome occurs despite the lack of any increase in strenuous physical exercise among participants. This pattern is confirmed by a recent meta-analysis,[96] and thus seems robust.

Based on this body of evidence, an expert panel convened by the US Centers for Disease Control and Prevention[97] recommended the following intervention tactics as the most likely to be effective:

1. Eliminate television from children's bedrooms
2. Reduce spontaneous media use in favor of planned media activities
3. Turn off the television while eating
4. Use school-based curricula to reduce children's screen time.

In the future, it will be important for research to better explicate the reasons why reductions in screen time lead to weight loss. Scholars have suggested that changes in energy intake, such as reduced snacking opportunities, as well as increases in low-level physical activity (eg, visiting friends outside the house instead of watching television at home), may underlie the effect. However, despite the lack of clarity about why reducing screen time helps to combat adiposity, it is clear that one way to reduce the obesity epidemic is to limit young people's time spent with media.

Limiting Unhealthy Food Advertising to Children

Although the first intervention strategy seeks to limit children's time spent with media, the second takes a different approach, seeking to reduce the amount of advertising for unhealthy foods that children encounter during their media use. The issue of unhealthy food marketing to children combines 2 distinct concerns: (1) the fairness of advertising to children, which applies to all merchandise; and (2) the propriety of promoting products to children that cannot be consumed safely in abundance. Youngsters do not comprehend the selling intent of commercials until at least 8 years of age, and they do not comprehend the persuasive bias inherent in advertising messages until several years later.[18,98,99] Before such recognition develops, children understand commercial claims and appeals as accurate, balanced, and truthful, failing to apply the skeptical eye of a more mature perspective. Based on this evidence, the American Psychological Association has concluded that all advertising targeted at young children is unfair because they lack the cognitive ability to defend against commercial persuasion.[100] Add in the consideration that most child-targeted food advertisements promote unhealthy products and it becomes obvious that food marketing to children is a serious public health issue.

Responding to public concern, the food industry established a self-regulatory effort known as the Children's Food and Beverage Advertising Initiative (CFBAI) in 2006.[101] With participation from more than a dozen of the nation's leading food conglomerates, the CFBAI is a pledge program in which each company commits to advertise foods to children only if they meet specified nutritional criteria for defining healthful products. For example, varying limits are placed on the amount of added fat, salt, and sugar

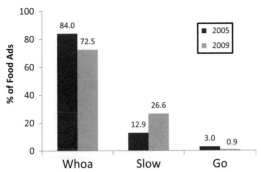

Fig. 3. Nutritional quality of foods advertised to children, before and after industry self-regulation. (*From* Kunkel D, McKinley C, Wright P. Assessing compliance with industry self-regulation of televised food marketing to children. Oakland (CA): Children Now; 2009; with permission.)

allowed for a product to qualify as healthy, thus making it permissible to advertise to children. Although the industry reports consistent evidence that companies generally fulfill their pledges,[101] independent research shows that the initiative has had only negligible effects in improving the nutritional quality of foods advertised to children.

In 2005, before industry self-regulation, 84% of all foods advertised on children's television programs were classified in the poorest nutritional category, according to standards used by the Department of Health and Human Services.[75] In 2009, several years following adoption of the CFBAI, that percentage had decreased only to 72.5%; nearly 3 out of 4 of the food products that met the industry's self-regulatory criteria for a healthy item were still nutritionally deficient (**Fig. 3**).

This result occurred for several reasons. Each participating company was allowed to use different nutritional standards to qualify their products as healthy for the purposes of the CFBAI, and many of their criteria were too lenient and self-serving.[102] In addition, more than one-quarter (28.7%) of food advertising to children originated with companies that chose not to participate in the CFBAI and hence were free to market whatever items they chose.[75] Industry self-regulation has achieved little in terms of addressing concerns about children's exposure to unhealthy food marketing, a finding confirmed by numerous studies using a broad range of nutritional measures.[103–105]

In 2011, the American Academy of Pediatrics issued a policy recommendation calling for a federal ban on junk food advertising during television programming viewed predominantly by young children.[30(p204)] Meanwhile, the food industry spent $51 million lobbying against regulation in the same year.[106] Although the industry asserts that First Amendment free speech protections prohibit any governmental restrictions on food advertising to children,[107] public health legal scholars have aggressively rebutted this position,[108,109] suggesting that a policy battle on this front may soon be on the horizon. One economics study[110] estimates that the impact of banning food advertisements on television would reduce the baseline rate of childhood obesity in the United States from 17% to somewhere in the range of 10.5% to 14.5%.

SUMMARY

Childhood obesity is viewed by many as the principal threat to the nation's public health. The malady currently afflicts more than 1 of every 6 American youth between the ages of 2 and 19 years,[111] each of whom faces a high probability of remaining obese into adulthood. The disease affects everyone in the country, given the tens of billions of dollars in obesity-related health care costs that are borne annually by the federal government. There is no single cause that accounts for the epidemic; it is a confluence of many factors that have converged to alter contemporary lifestyles, with media a prominent factor in this problem. To reverse the prevalence of childhood obesity will require significant shifts in many aspects of children's everyday environments. Reducing the time children spend with media, as well as reducing the number of advertisements for unhealthy food products in child-targeted media, are key goals in the battle.

Progress to date has been limited on both fronts. Population norms for children's media use continue at high levels.[25,27] Food industry efforts at reform have been tepid,[112] and governmental action has also been lacking.[113] To obtain sufficient societal awareness, concern, and support to overcome the epidemic requires changes on the scale of a social movement similar to the shift that has been accomplished in attitudes and regulations toward smoking and tobacco.[114] Although that challenge is daunting, it is nonetheless critical for maintaining the health of future generations.

REFERENCES

1. Ogden CL, Carroll MD, Curtin LR, et al. Prevalence of high body mass index in US children and adolescents, 2007-2008. JAMA 2010;303(3):242–9.
2. Freedman DS, Mei Z, Srinivasan SR, et al. Cardiovascular risk factors and excess adiposity among overweight children and adolescents: the Bogalusa Heart Study. J Pediatr 2007;150(1):12–17, e2.
3. Whitlock EP, Williams SB, Gold R, et al. Screening and interventions for childhood overweight: a summary of evidence for the US Preventive Services Task Force. Pediatrics 2005;116(1):e125–44.
4. Han JC, Lawlor DA, Kimm SY. Childhood obesity. Lancet 2010;375(9727): 1737–48.
5. Sutherland ER. Obesity and asthma. Immunol Allergy Clin North Am 2008;28(3): 589–602.
6. Taylor ED, Theim KR, Mirch MC, et al. Orthopedic complications of overweight in children and adolescents. Pediatrics 2006;117(6):2167–74.
7. Dietz W. Health consequences of obesity in youth: childhood predictors of adult disease. Pediatrics 1998;101:518–25.
8. Swartz MB, Puhl R. Childhood obesity: a societal problem to solve. Obes Rev 2003;4(1):57–71.
9. Whitaker RC, Wright JA, Pepe MS, et al. Predicting obesity in young adulthood from childhood and parental obesity. N Engl J Med 1997;37(13):869–73.
10. Serdula MK, Ivery D, Coates RJ, et al. Do obese children become obese adults? A review of the literature. Prev Med 1993;22:167–77.
11. Dietz WH Jr, Gortmaker SL. Do we fatten our children at the television set? Obesity and television viewing in children and adolescents. Pediatrics 1985; 75(5):807–12.
12. Gortmaker SL, Must A, Sobol AM, et al. Television viewing as a cause of increasing obesity among children in the United States, 1986-1990. Arch Pediatr Adolesc Med 1996;150(4):356–62.
13. Lobstein T, Baur L, Uauy R. Obesity in children and young people: a crisis in public health. Obs Rev 2004;5(s1):4–85.
14. Bar-Or O, Foreyt J, Bouchard C, et al. Physical activity, genetic and nutritional consideration in childhood weight management. Med Sci Sports Exerc 1998; 30:2–10.

15. Chen J, Kennedy C. Television viewing and children's health. J Soc Pediatr Nurs 2001;1:35–6.
16. Vandewater E, Cummings H. Media use and childhood obesity. In: Calvert S, Wilson B, editors. The handbook of children, media, and development. West Sussex (United Kingdom): Blackwell Publishing; 2008. p. 355–80.
17. Lobstein T, Dibb S. Evidence of a possible link between obesogenic food advertising and child overweight. Obes Rev 2005;6:203–8.
18. Kunkel D, Castonguay J. Children and advertising: content, comprehension, and consequences. In: Singer DG, Singer JL, editors. Handbook of children and the media. 2nd edition. Thousand Oaks (CA): Sage Publications; 2012. p. 95–418.
19. Powell LM, Schermbeck RM, Szczypka G, et al. Trends in the nutritional content of television food advertisements seen by children in the United States. Arch Pediatr Adolesc Med 2011;165(12):1078–86.
20. Rudd Center for Food Policy and Obesity. Trends in television food advertising to you people: 2010 update. New Haven (CT): Yale University; 2011.
21. Chester J, Montgomery KC. Interactive food & beverage marketing: targeting children and youth in the digital age. The Berkeley Media Studies Group web site. Available at: http://digitalads.org/documents/digiMarketingFull.pdf. 2007. Accessed February 1, 2012.
22. Culp J, Bell R, Cassaday D. Characteristics of food industry websites and advergames targeting children. J Nutr Educ Behav 2010;42(3):197–201.
23. Jain A. Temptations in cyberspace: new battlefields in childhood obesity. Health Aff 2010;29(3):425–9.
24. Institute of Medicine (IOM). Food marketing to children and youth: threat or opportunity? Washington, DC: National Academies Press; 2006.
25. Rideout VJ, Foehr UG, Roberts DF. Generation M2: media in the lives of 8- to 18-year-olds. Menlo Park (CA): The Henry J Kaiser Family Foundation; 2010.
26. Vandewater E, Lee S. Measuring children's media use in the digital age: issues and challenges. Am Behav Sci 2009;52(8):1152–76.
27. Vandewater E, Rideout V, Wartella E, et al. Digital childhood: electronic media and technology use among infants, toddlers, and preschoolers. Pediatrics 2007;199:1006–15.
28. Birch L, Parker L, Burns A. Early childhood obesity prevention policies. Washington, DC: The National Academies Press; 2011.
29. Rideout VJ, Vandewater E, Wartella E. Zero to six: electronic media in the lives of infants, toddlers and preschoolers. Menlo Park (CA): The Henry J Kaiser Family Foundation; 2003.
30. American Academy of Pediatrics, Council on Communications and Media. Media use by children younger than two years. Pediatrics 2011;128:1040–5.
31. Christakis D, Zimmerman F, DiGiuseppe D, et al. Early television exposure and subsequent attentional problems in children. Pediatrics 2004;113(4):708–13.
32. Common sense media. Zero to eight: children's media use in America; common sense media Web site. Available at: http://www.commonsensemedia.org/sites/default/files/research/zerotoeightfinal2011.pdf. 2011. Accessed February 1, 2012.
33. Foehr U. Media multitasking among American youth: prevalence, predictors, and pairings. Menlo Park (CA): The Henry J Kaiser Family Foundation; 2006.
34. Bushman B, Huesmann L. Effects of violent media on aggression. In: Singer D, Singer J, editors. Handbook of children and the media. 2nd edition. Thousand Oaks (CA): Sage Publications; 2012. p. 249–72.

35. Collins R, Elliott M, Berry S, et al. Watching sex on TV affects adolescent initiation of sexual intercourse. Pediatrics 2004;114(3):e280–9.

36. Signorielli N. Television's gender role images and contribution to stereotyping: past present future. In: Singer D, Singer J, editors. Handbook of children and the media. 2nd edition. Thousand Oaks (CA): Sage Publications; 2012. p. 321–40.

37. Asamen J, Berry G. Television, children, and multicultural awareness: comprehending the medium in a complex multimedia society. In: Singer D, Singer J, editors. Handbook of children and the media. 2nd edition. Thousand Oaks (CA): Sage Publications; 2012. p. 363–78.

38. Gable S, Chang Y, Krull J. Television watching and frequency of family meals are predictive of overweight onset and persistence in a national sample of school-aged children. J Am Diet Assoc 2007;107(1):53–61.

39. Sisson SB, Broyles ST, Baker BL, et al. Screen time, physical activity, and overweight in U.S. youth: National Survey of Children's Health 2003. J Adolesc Health 2010;47(3):309–11.

40. te Velde S, De Bourdeaudhuij I, Thorsdottir I, et al. Patterns in sedentary and exercise behaviors and associations with overweight in 9–14-year-old boys and girls - a cross-sectional study. BMC Public Health 2007;7(16):1–9.

41. Utter J, Scragg R, Schaaf D. Associations between television viewing and consumption of commonly advertised foods among New Zealand children and young adolescents. Public Health Nutr 2006;9(5):606–12.

42. Zimmerman FJ, Bell JF. Associations of television content type and obesity in children. Am J Public Health 2010;100:334–40.

43. Nunez-Smith M, Wolf E, Huang H, et al. Media and child and adolescent health: a systematic review. San Francisco (CA): Common Sense Media; 2008.

44. Salmon J, Jorna M, Hume C, et al. A translational research intervention to reduce screen behaviours and promote physical activity among children: Switch-2-Activity. Health Promot Int 2011;26(3):311–21.

45. McMurray RG, Harrel JS, Deng S, et al. The influence of physical activity, socioeconomic status, and ethnicity on the weight status of adolescents. Obes Res 2000;8(2):130–9.

46. Vandewater E, Shim M, Caplovitz A. Linking obesity and activity level with children's television and video game use. J Adolesc 2004;27(1):71–85.

47. Wake M, Hesketh K, Waters E. Television, computer use and body mass index in Australian primary school children. J Paediatr Child Health 2003;39(2):130–4.

48. Kautiainen S, Koivusilta L, Lintonen T, et al. Use of information and communication technology and prevalence of overweight and obesity among adolescents. Int J Obes (Lond) 2005;29(8):925–33.

49. Rey-Lopez JP, Vicente-Rodriguez G, Biosca M, et al. Sedentary behaviour and obesity development in children and adolescents. Nutr Metab Cardiovasc Dis 2008;18(3):242–51.

50. Pate RR. Physically active video gaming: an effective strategy for obesity prevention? Arch Pediatr Adolesc Med 2008;162(9):895–6.

51. Graf DL, Pratt LV, Hester CN, et al. Playing active video games increases energy expenditure in children. Pediatrics 2009;124(2):534–40.

52. Daley A. Can exergaming contribute to improving physical activity levels and health outcomes in children? Pediatrics 2009;124:763–74.

53. Robinson TN. Reducing children's television viewing to prevent obesity: a randomized controlled trial. J Am Med Assoc 1999;282(16):1561–7.

54. Council on Communications and Media. Children, adolescents, obesity and the media. Elk Grove Village (IL): American Academy of Pediatrics; 2011.

55. Nelson MC, Neumark-Sztainer D, Hannan PJ, et al. Longitudinal and secular trends in physical activity and sedentary behavior during adolescence. Pediatrics 2006;118(6):e1627–34.

56. Hardy LL, Bass SL, Booth ML. Changes in sedentary behavior among adolescent girls: a 2.5-year prospective cohort study. J Adolesc Health 2007;40(2): 158–65.

57. Burdette HL, Whitaker RC. A national study of neighborhood safety, outdoor play, television viewing, and obesity in preschool children. Pediatrics 2005; 116(3):657–62.

58. Taveras EM, Field AE, Berkey CS, et al. Longitudinal relationship between television viewing and leisure-time physical activity during adolescence. Pediatrics 2007;119(2):e314–25.

59. Melkevik O, Torsheim T, Iannotti RJ, et al. Is spending time in screen-based sedentary behaviors associated with less physical activity: a cross national investigation. Int J Behav Nutr Phys Act 2010;7:46–56.

60. Dowda M, Brown W, McIver K, et al. Policies and characteristics of the preschool environment and physical activity of young children. Pediatrics 2009;123(2):e261–6.

61. Bower J, Hales D, Tate D, et al. The childcare environment and children's physical activity. Am J Prev Med 2008;34(1):23–9.

62. Dowda M, Pate R, Trost S, et al. Influences of preschool policies and practices on children's physical activity. J Community Health 2004;29(3):183–96.

63. Anderson S, Economos C, Must A. Active play and screen time in US children aged 4 to 11 years in relation to sociodemographic and weight status characteristics: a nationally representative cross-sectional analysis. BMC Public Health 2008;8:366–79.

64. Holt D, Ippolito P, Desrochers D, et al. Children's exposure to TV advertising in 1977 and 2004: information for the obesity debate. Federal Trade Commission Web site. Available at: http://www.ftc.gov/os/2007/06/cabecolor.pdf. 2007. Accessed February 12, 2012.

65. Kunkel D, McIlrath M. Message content in advertising to children. In: Palmer EL, Young BM, editors. The faces of televisual media: teaching violence, selling to children. Mahwah (NJ): Lawrence Erlbaum; 2003. p. 287–300.

66. Palmer E, Carpenter CF. Food and beverage marketing to children and youth: trends and issues. Media Psychol 2006;8(2):165–90.

67. Federal Trade Commission. Marketing food to children and adolescents: a review of industry expenditures, activities, and self-regulation. Federal Trade Commission web site. Available at: http://www.ftc.gov/opa/2008/07/foodmkting.shtm. Accessed February 11, 2012.

68. Story M, French S. Food advertising and marketing directed at children and adolescents in the US. Int J Behav Nutr Phys Act 2004;1(3):1–17.

69. Schwartz MB, Vartanian LR, Wharton CM, et al. Examining the nutritional quality of breakfast cereals marketed to children. J Am Diet Assoc 2008; 108(4):702–5.

70. Gantz W, Schwartz N, Angelini J, et al. Food for thought: television food advertising to children in the United States. Menlo Park (CA): The Henry J Kaiser Family Foundation; 2007.

71. Stitt C, Kunkel D. Food advertising during children's television programming on broadcast and cable channels. Health Commun 2008;23:573–84.

72. Alvy LM, Calvert SL. Food marketing on popular children's websites: a content analysis. J Am Diet Assoc 2008;108(4):710–3.

73. Lingas E, Dorfman L, Bukofzer E. Nutrition content of food and beverage products on web sites popular with children. Am J Public Health 2009;99(7):1–10.

74. Kunkel D, Wilcox B. Children and media policy: historical perspectives and current practices. In: Singer DG, Singer JL, editors. Handbook of children and the media. 2nd edition. Thousand Oaks (CA): Sage Publications; 2012. p. 569–94.

75. Kunkel D, McKinley C, Wright P. Assessing compliance with industry self-regulation of televised food marketing to children. Oakland (CA): Children Now; 2009.

76. Simply Zesty. Trends in in-game advertising. Simply Zesty Web site. Available at: http://www.simplyzesty.com/advertising-and-marketing/advertising/trends-ingame-advertising/. 2010. Accessed February 13, 2012.

77. Montgomery KC, Chester J. Interactive food and beverage marketing: targeting adolescents in the digital age. J Adolesc Health 2009;45:S18–29.

78. Public Citizen. School commercialism: high costs, low revenues. Public Citizen Web site. Available at: www.citizen.org; 2012. Accessed February 12, 2012.

79. Linn S. Consuming kids: the hostile takeover of childhood. New York: The New Press; 2004.

80. Schor JB. Born to buy: the commercialized child and the new consumer culture. New York: Scribner; 2004.

81. Thomas SG. Buy, buy baby: how consumer culture manipulates parents and harms young minds. New York: Houghton Mifflin; 2007.

82. Harrison K. Is "fat free" good for me? A panel study of television viewing and children's nutritional knowledge and reasoning. Health Commun 2005;17:117–32.

83. Signorielli N, Lears M. Television and children's conceptions of nutrition: unhealthy messages. Health Commun 1997;4:245–57.

84. Signorielli N, Staples J. Television and children's conceptions of nutrition. Health Commun 1997;9:289–301.

85. Gunter B, Oates C, Blades M. Advertising to children on TV: content, impact, and regulation. Mahwah (NJ): Lawrence Erlbaum Associates; 2005.

86. Valkenburg PM, Buijzen M. Identifying determinants of young children's brand awareness: television, parents, and peers. Appl Dev Psychol 2005;26:456–68.

87. Buijzen M, Schuurman J, Bomhof E. Associations between children's television advertising exposure and their food consumption patterns: a household diary survey study. Appetite 2008;50(2):231–9.

88. O'Dougherty M, Story M, Stang J. Observations of parent-child co-shoppers in supermarkets: children's involvement in food selections, parental yielding, and refusal strategies. J Nutr Educ Behav 2006;38:183–8.

89. Wilson G, Wood K. The influence of children on parental purchases during supermarket shopping. Int J Consum Stud 2004;28(4):329–36.

90. Dotson MJ, Hyatt EM. Major influence factors in children's consumer socialization. J Consum Market 2005;22(1):35–43.

91. Dennison B, Russo T, Burdick P, et al. An intervention to reduce television viewing by preschool children. Arch Pediatr Adolesc Med 2004;158(2):170–6.

92. Epstein L, Roemmich J, Robinson J, et al. A randomized trial of the effects of reducing television viewing and computer use on body mass index in young children. Arch Pediatr Adolesc Med 2008;162(3):239–45.

93. Epstein L, Paluch R, Gordy C, et al. Decreasing sedentary behaviors in treating pediatric obesity. Arch Pediatr Adolesc Med 2000;154(3):220–6.

94. Gortmaker SL, Peterson K, Wiecha J, et al. Reducing obesity via a school-based interdisciplinary intervention among youth: planet health. Arch Pediatr Adolesc Med 1999;153:409–18.

95. Robinson T, Borzekowski D. Effects of the smart classroom curriculum to reduce child and family screen time. J Comm 2006;56(1):1–26.
96. Wahi G, Parkin P, Beyene J, et al. A systematic review and meta-analysis of randomized controlled trials. Arch Pediatr Adolesc Med 2011;165(11):979–86.
97. Jordan A, Robinson T. Children, television viewing, and weight status: summary and recommendations from an expert panel meeting. Ann Am Acad Pol Soc Sci 2008;615:119–32.
98. Kunkel D. Mismeasurement of children's understanding of the persuasive intent of advertising. J Child Media 2010;4:109–17.
99. Wright P, Friestad M, Boush D. The development of marketplace persuasion knowledge in children, adolescents, and young adults. J Public Policy Mark 2005;24(2):222–33.
100. Kunkel D, Wilcox BL, Cantor J, et al. Report of the APA task force on advertising and children. American Psychological Association Web site. Available at: http://www.apa.org/pi/families/resources/advertising-children.pdf. 2004. Accessed February 13, 2012.
101. Kolish E, Hernandez M, Blanchard K. The Children's Food and Beverage Advertising Initiative in action: a report on compliance and implementation during 2010 and a five year retrospective: 2006-2011. Arlington (VA): Council of Better Business Bureaus; 2011.
102. Wootan M, Batada A, Balkus O. Report card on food-marketing policies. Center for Science in the Public Interest Web site. Available at: http://cspinet.org/new/pdf/marketingreportcard.pdf. Accessed February 13, 2012.
103. Batada A, Seitz M, Wootan M, et al. Nine out of 10 food advertisements shown during Saturday morning children's programming are for foods high in fat, sodium, or added sugars, or low in nutrients. J Am Diet Assoc 2008;108:673–8.
104. Harris J, Weinberg M, Schwartz M, et al. Trends in television food advertising: progress in reducing unhealthy marketing to young people? Rudd Center for Food Policy and Obesity Web site. Available at: http://www.yaleruddcenter.org/resources/upload/docs/what/reports/RuddReport_TVFoodAdvertising_2.10.pdf. 2010. Accessed February 13, 2012.
105. Powell L, Szczypka G, Chaloupka F. Trends in exposure to television food advertisements among children and adolescents in the United States. Arch Pediatr Adolesc Med 2011;164(9):1–9.
106. Sunlight Foundation. Food and media companies lobby to weaken guidelines on marketing food to children. Sunlight Foundation Web site. Available at: http://reporting.sunlightfoundation.com/2011/Food_and_media_companies_lobby/. 2011. Accessed February 13. 2012.
107. Jaffe DL. Food marketing: can "voluntary" government restrictions improve children's health? Testimony on behalf of the Association of National Advertisers for the Subcommittee on Commerce, Manufacturing and Trade and the Subcommittee on Health House Energy and Commerce Committee. Washington, DC: House Energy and Commerce Committee; 2011. Available at: http://energycommerce.house.gov/hearings/hearingdetail.aspx?NewsID=8973. Accessed February 13, 2012.
108. Graff S, Kunkel D, Mermin S. Government can regulate food advertising to children because cognitive research shows that it is inherently misleading. Health Aff 2012;31(2):392–8.
109. Harris J, Graff S. Protecting young people from junk food advertising: implications of psychological research for First Amendment law. Am J Public Health 2012;102:214–22.

110. Veerman JL, Van Beeck E, Barendregt J, et al. By how much would limiting TV food advertising reduce childhood obesity? Eur J Public Health 2009;19(4): 365–9.

111. Ogden CL, Carroll MD, Kit BK, et al. Prevalence of obesity and trends in body mass index among US children and adolescents, 1999-2010. JAMA 2012; 307(5):E1–8.

112. Kraak V, Story M, Wartella E, et al. Industry progress to market a healthful diet to American children and adolescents. Am J Prev Med 2011;41(3):322–33.

113. Brescoll VL, Kersh R, Brownell KD. Assessing the feasibility and impact of federal childhood obesity policies. Ann Am Acad Pol Soc Sci 2008;615:178–94.

114. Klein JD, Dietz W. Childhood obesity: the new tobacco. Health Aff 2010;29(3): 388–92.

Body Image, Eating Disorders, and the Relationship to Adolescent Media Use

Carson A. Benowitz-Fredericks, BA, Kaylor Garcia, BA,
Meredith Massey, EdM, Brintha Vasagar, MD, MPH,
Dina L.G. Borzekowski, EdD*

KEYWORDS

- Anorexia • Bulimia • Internet • Television • Weight concerns • Body dissatisfaction

KEY POINTS

- Historically and currently, media messages around body shape and size emphasize the importance of being below-average weight for women and hypermuscular for men.
- The media messages around physical appearance are not realistic for most and lead to body dissatisfaction for adolescents.
- Interventions designed to mitigate the influence of negative media messages on adolescents' body image are presented; however, most have shown limited success.

Although in flux throughout life, an individual's body image begins to solidify in early adolescence.[1] The construct of body image is multidimensional, and includes cognitive, affective, evaluative, and behavioral aspects of physical appearance.[1,2] Evaluative or attitudinal body image changes with life experiences as individuals assimilate sociocultural body ideals and determines their own physical self-satisfaction.[1,2]

The development of body image is of particular interest, because extreme physical and cognitive changes occur during this period. During puberty, children gain 50% of their adult body weight, and girls experience an increase in body fat and widening of the hips.[3,4] With Western culture favoring a thin physique, these changes can pull girls farther from the ideal body shape. Puberty does the opposite for boys; adolescent boys experience changes that bring them closer to the cultural ideal of a large, muscular man.[4,5] These gender differences arise at 13 to 15 years of age, with girls experiencing increased body dissatisfaction and boys experiencing decreased body dissatisfaction.[6]

Department of Health, Behavior and Society, Johns Hopkins Bloomberg School of Public Health, 624 North Broadway, #745, Baltimore, MD 21205, USA
* Corresponding author.
E-mail address: dborzeko@jhsph.edu

Pediatr Clin N Am 59 (2012) 693–704
doi:10.1016/j.pcl.2012.03.017
0031-3955/12/$ – see front matter © 2012 Elsevier Inc. All rights reserved.

Cognitively, adolescence is also accompanied by increased awareness of societal norms and values surrounding physical appearance and relationships.[3,7,8] Concurrently, the circulation of gonadal hormones can increase sexual interest and place further importance on body image.[3] Adolescent dating behaviors and notions of physical desirability are heavily guided by peers, families, and media.[1,4,8] Adolescent girls often derive self-esteem from their physical appearance. In this context, thinness is important. Adolescent girls associate thinness with beauty, popularity, and successful dating relationships.[7,8] Adolescent boys also rate female thinness as an important factor in determining attractiveness and dateability. This scrutiny often leads to feelings of inadequacy in body shape, and increased interaction between genders has been positively associated with body dissatisfaction.[8]

Based on a biopsychosocial model, body dissatisfaction, or negative evaluation of one's own body compared with an ideal body, is modulated by multiple factors.[3,7] From a biologic standpoint, increased body mass index has been correlated with increased body dissatisfaction, although this varies by gender.[1,9] Race may also play a role, with studies showing that Caucasian adolescents report more body dissatisfaction than African American adolescents.[3] Psychological factors include low self-esteem, which is one of the strongest risk factors for body dissatisfaction. Adolescents who create strict evaluative criteria for success and strive for perfection may never realize their body ideal, and may remain perpetually dissatisfied with their bodies.[9]

Sociocultural factors related to body image can promote unrealistic standards of physical appearance, which are unattainable for most adolescents.[9] Socially, peers are an important influence. Weight-related teasing and encouragement to lose weight may contribute to body dissatisfaction.[9,10] Additionally, girls who compare their bodies with those of peers are more likely to report negative body image.[10] Parents, too, have a strong influence. Negative body image is correlated to parental complaints about their own weight and mothers' comments about their daughters' weights.[10] In girls, a drive for thinness, or the willingness to alter one's body to meet the social ideal of physical attractiveness, was correlated with parental encouragement to lose weight and the mothers' dieting behaviors.

Most adolescents who develop body dissatisfaction do not experience clinical manifestations, but, in some, eating disorders may develop.[3,11] Aspects of body image, such as low self-esteem and self-oriented perfectionism, lead adolescents to pursue unattainable physical appearances and have been suggested as prerequisites for the development of eating disorders.[7,12] Some adolescents develop dichotomous thinking patterns that can lead to eating disorders. Individuals with this type of thinking believe that higher-order goals, such as happiness, are unattainable without first reaching lower-order goals, such as losing weight. This type of thinking places increased emphasis on the relentless pursuit of unrealistic body ideals in an effort to achieve happiness and wellness.[12]

Using *Diagnostic and Statistical Manual of Mental Disorders* (Fourth Edition) (DSM-IV) criteria, the lifetime prevalence estimates of anorexia nervosa, bulimia nervosa, and binge eating disorder in women in Europe and the United States are 0.9%, 1.5%, and 3.5%, respectively; men in the same study had prevalence estimates of 0.3%, 0.5%, and 3.5%.[13] In Australia, cross-sectional surveys have shown that the prevalence of disordered eating behaviors, such as binging, purging, and strict dieting, more than doubled between 1995 and 2005; this increase was attributed to increased public preoccupation with weight.[14] Prevalence figures, however, are difficult to compare because they vary greatly among countries and studies because of sociocultural differences in baseline values and variations in study methods.[15] For example, the lifetime prevalence of anorexia nervosa is 1.2% in Sweden, but only between 0.5% and 1% in the United States.[15,16] These rates may also underestimate disordered eating, because subthreshold disordered eating is not included in these values.[15]

The incidence of eating disorders is difficult to measure, because it is often limited to those who seek medical treatment. In Europe, the incidence of anorexia cases increased from the 1950s through the 1970s and stabilized thereafter. However, whether this is because of true changes in incidence within the population or simply fluctuations in the reporting of cases is unclear.[16–18] Although the incidence of bulimia in the United Kingdom between 1988 and 1993 increased threefold before finally peaking in 1996 and declining until 2000, British media coverage of Princess Diana's struggle with bulimia during the 1990s is hypothesized to have led to a rise in reported cases of bulimia despite no actual increase in incidence within the population.[18] Studies in the United States also show an increase in incidence of bulimia over the 20th century, but the trend for anorexia continues to be debated without any clear or reliable pattern.[13]

By 13 years of age, eating disorders become more common in girls. By 15 years of age, girls are three times more likely to display disordered eating than boys.[7] This finding may be because adolescent girls tend to have more negative body images than adolescent boys. Both anorexia nervosa and bulimia nervosa have a peak incidence at 16 to 17 years of age.[9]

MEDIA MESSAGES ABOUT APPEARANCE
Magazines

Throughout history, women's magazines have emphasized the importance of appearance. In contrast to men's magazines, women's magazines constantly offer weight loss messages and equate beauty with positive life outcomes.[19] Often these magazines present incompatible messages. For instance, in *Seventeen*, models featured in both articles and advertisements have extremely slim body types, whereas the text often advises readers to think outside of standard conceptions of beauty ideals.[20] One study of magazine covers found that 61% offered conflicting headlines, such as "Trim Your Thighs in 3 Weeks" and "Ice Cream Extravaganza." However, magazines vary; in one study, fashion magazines (eg, *Glamour*) averaged 14.8 articles over 6 months on weight reduction compared with 11.2 and 5.7 articles in traditional (eg, *Good Housekeeping*) and modern (eg, *New Woman*) magazines, respectively.[19]

Messages about body image also differ depending on the magazine's target audience. Among cover models featured on *Ebony*, a magazine targeting African American readers, 76.4% were average weight, and just 5.7% were underweight.[21] Analyses of magazines targeting gay and lesbian readers have found messages about hypermuscularity in the gay men's magazines and more diverse body representations in the lesbian magazines.[22,23] In *Men's Health* and *Men's Fitness*, nearly all (>95%) of the featured models had extremely low levels of body fat and most (>78%) were considered very muscular.[24]

On-Screen Media: TV and Movies

In a study of cartoons over 9 decades, researchers found that body weight and physical attractiveness were inversely related. Female characters were much more likely to be physically attractive than male characters. Overweight characters were three times as likely to be characterized as less smart and less competent than their underweight and normal weight counterparts. Attractive characters were happier and more prosocial.[25]

In television programs for preadolescents, lead characters tend to be underweight, Story lines and character interactions frequently focus on an idealize female body shape. Non–ideal-shaped preadolescent girls are often cast as Goths or bullies.[26] In programs for adolescent audiences, the highest percentage of characters fall into the normal weight range, followed by those on the thinner side. Heavyset or obese characters are rare or nonexistent. However, 40% of African American female characters are above-average weight compared with 12.7% of Caucasian women.[27]

In soap operas and situation comedies (sitcoms), programming genres frequently watched by young audiences, characters tend to be thinner than the average population.[28,29] This finding is especially pronounced in soap operas, with half of the characters of low to low-average weight.[29] A third of female characters on sitcoms, compared with 25% of the general population, are of below-average weight. Additionally, these women receive more positive comments about their appearance and are involved in more romantic relationships than heavier characters.[28] Although overweight men in sitcoms do not receive negative comments about their appearance, they were more likely to make self-deprecating statements.[30] African American women, who are underrepresented in most television genres, appear more frequently in music videos; here, they are typically underweight and extremely sexualized.[31]

In children's movies, there is an average of 8.7 body image–related messages. In a 2004 content analysis of children's books and videos, approximately 60% of the videos focused on female thinness whereas 32% of videos emphasized male muscularity.[32] Disney animated movies portrayed almost half of villains as overweight compared with 10% of heroes. These differences were especially pronounced among female characters, because male characters had more homogenous bodies.[33] Action movies typically emphasize hypermuscularity for boys and men. Approximately three-fourths of characters tend to be muscular, and these muscular characters have more appealing traits and are involved in more romantic partnerships.[34]

New Media: Video Games and the Internet

Video game representations, at least during game play, seem to offer more realistic body image messages for both genders. For women, female characters closely resembled the proportions of average fit women, with breast size being the only significant difference.[35] Male characters were blockier and not well defined, with less emphasis on muscularity than is found in other media sources.[36]

A new analysis of YouTube has found that videos with fat-stigmatizing content (in the videos, titles, or commentary) are often produced by or geared toward Caucasian men. Women constituted only 7.7% of antagonists but one-third of victims. Men were 11.5 times more likely to be aggressors than women, but only 1.7 times more likely to be victims. These trends seem more severe than those seen in other media.[37]

The Internet contains easily accessible Web sites focusing on anorexia and bulimia, known as e-Ana and e-Mia Web sites. Interactive features allow users to interact and support each other through poetry and artwork, building a social system for these teens who otherwise struggle to relate to peers. Although 30% of sites had accessories like food calculators to aid visitors in managing weight, more common messages are about strategies to continue the pro–eating disorder (pro-ED) thinking and behaviors. However, approximately 38% of these sites provide information and links to help users recover from the eating disorders.[38]

THE RELATIONSHIP AMONG MEDIA USE, BODY IMAGE PERCEPTIONS, AND EATING DISORDERS
Correlational Studies

As global obesity rates rise, researchers have observed that greater media use during childhood and adolescence is associated with higher weight status and poorer fitness in adulthood.[39] However, evidence exists of a media-use relationship on other end of the scale. Exposure to certain media seems to be significantly associated with body dissatisfaction, vulnerability to heightened weight-control, and dieting disorders.

A large longitudinal study following more than 2500 girls in middle and high school from Minnesota showed that heavy readers of magazines were twice as likely to engage in disordered weight-control behaviors.[40] A Spanish study following 2862 girls and women for 18 months, ranging in age from 12 to 21 years, showed doubled odds for incident eating disorders among those who frequently read girls' magazines and listened to radio programs.[41] A significant positive correlation between hours spent watching music videos and importance of appearance and weight concerns was found when looking at a population of ninth-grade girls from California.[42] A longitudinal study of lower-middle and middle income communities in Midwestern states found that among preteen girls, greater overall television viewing time predicted thinner shapes 1 year later.[43] Of particular potential potency are pro-ED Web sites (eg, pro-ana, pro-mia). One study found that users of pro-ED sites seem to have higher levels of body dissatisfaction and eating disturbances.[44] Another assessment of 1291 users of pro-ED sites found that heavier use of the Web sites was associated with higher scores on measures of eating disorders, more extreme weight loss behaviors, and a greater likelihood of hospitalization.[45]

In terms of general media exposures, boys and girls may be affected differently. A cross-sectional study of 828 adolescents showed that both messages encouraging muscularity and those promoting thinness predicted compulsive exercise in boys, whereas girls were only susceptible to messages about thinness.[46] In a survey of 353 undergraduates from a large Western state college in the United States, women experienced more symptoms of disordered eating than did men. The researchers also found that media, perfectionism, and self-esteem were related to women's eating disorders, whereas only media and perfectionism related to the men's.[47] Additional specialized channels have been identified, including video gaming magazines, which were associated with a drive for muscularity in White (but not African American) boys.[48] Gay and bisexual adolescents and college-aged boys may be more vulnerable to media influence on body image, whereas lesbian and bisexual girls may be less so.[49,50]

Not all media effects are detrimental, however. In a sample of 11,606 boys and girls, desire to resemble media figures was associated with higher physical activity levels.[51] Moreover, a forthcoming study on identification with media figures showed that women exposed to a favorite celebrity or a thin model with whom they perceived similarity felt better, not worse, about their bodies.[52]

Experimental Studies

A meta-analysis of 25 experimental studies showed that, especially for girls younger than 19 years, viewing images of thin models produced a more negative body image.[53] An experiment involving 145 college women showed that exposure to thin-ideal magazine images not only lowered self-esteem but increased symptoms of eating disorders.[54] Compared with fashion-site controls, controlled exposure to a mock pro-ED Web site induced lower social self-esteem and appearance self-efficacy, and a greater negative affect in exposed women. In addition, those in the exposure group perceived themselves as heavier and were more compelled to exercise and think about their weight.[55] Pro-ED sites proved to be a potent pill; female college students exposed to the sites for 1.5 hours showed a 1-week postexposure decline in caloric intake from 12,167 to 9697 calories, and reported making use of techniques described on the Web sites.[56]

The experimental literature hints at differential vulnerabilities. In one study, subjects already identified as either restrained or unrestrained eaters were exposed to advertisements featuring thin models or nonfigures. Exposure to the model images led to reports of more favorable self-image and social self-esteem in restrained eaters, whereas unrestrained eaters reported lower appearance self-esteem score.[57] In a 15-month longitudinal experiment, girls who had higher levels of body dissatisfaction and less social support at baseline, when subjected to increased exposure to fashion magazines, exhibited a significantly greater likelihood of further body dissatisfaction, dieting, and bulimic symptoms at experiment's end compared with those less vulnerable. Meanwhile, the study population as a whole showed no effect from level of magazine exposure.[58] Likewise, exposure to appearance-centric commercials triggered more body image changes and thoughts of dietary restraint in patients with eating disorders but had no effect on those without.[59]

POTENTIAL EXPLANATIONS OF THE RELATIONSHIP AMONG MEDIA USE, BODY IMAGE, AND EATING DISORDERS

The strong influence of media on adolescents occurs not only directly but also indirectly through creation and reinforcement of social norms at all levels of society. Although the effects of negative or unrealistic media images differ between groups (eg, girls vs boys),[60–62] no group seems to be entirely immune. In fact, media images are so pervasive that they can be said to affect the whole of society, with the most vulnerable members of any particular group exhibiting the most negative effects of media influence.[63]

Understanding of media influence on body image and eating disorders relies largely on sociocultural modeling. Media effectively transmits and reinforces certain sociocultural messages, including a thin-ideal body image for girls, hypermuscularity for boys, strict gender role reinforcement, and primacy of appearance as a factor for success.[64–66] Although these messages are spread through various social mechanisms, media has been the main subject of research because of its pervasiveness and power at all levels of society.

Media effects seem to be cumulative in that, in most cases, greater exposure to overt messages regarding appearance predicts internalization of these social ideals.[67,68] After repeated exposure to media content, viewers may internalize media portrayals of unrealistic ideals. In this way, the ideal image becomes normative.[65,67,69] Social comparison theory, in which individuals develop a self-evaluation in comparison with others, has also been used to explain media influence in this area. Typically, adolescents make an "upward" comparison between themselves and ultrathin or hypermuscled media models, resulting in feelings of body dissatisfaction, lower self-esteem, and unhealthy eating behaviors.[66,70,71]

The relationship between media influence and body image usually involves small to medium effect sizes.[72,73] The relationship is complicated by a variety of moderating and mediating factors. Mediators of media effect include internalization of the thin-ideal, social comparison, and activation of the thin-ideal schema.[74] Other factors, such as social support from peers and family and age, also have been shown to have a significant impact. Recently, weight/shape-related self-ideal discrepancy and self-concept clarity have been proposed as additional mechanisms involved in the relationship between media and body image.[69,75]

Family and peers can alter the relationship between media messages and body dissatisfaction. Family influences, early in childhood and into adolescence, set the stage for susceptibility to body dissatisfaction and eating disorders.[76,77] Parents and siblings transmit and reinforce social messages, and act as role models for body image attitudes and eating behavior. Although mothers and fathers have a different influence on girls versus boys, positive family relationships seem to somewhat insulate both genders from negative messages.[76,78] Entering adolescence, peers become more significant in shaping body image and eating patterns. According to the presumed influence model, media effects on adolescents may be greater because adolescents perceive their family and peers to also be influenced by media messages.[79–82]

Personal characteristics may also affect adolescents' body satisfaction and susceptibility to the influence of media images, although more research is needed in this area. Individuals whose self-schemas included a divergence between their actual body type and their ideal body type are more susceptible to body dissatisfaction and the influence of negative media messages.[83] Experimental studies have found that only "high internalizers" showed a large increase in body dissatisfaction after viewing ultrathin models.[83] Additionally, factors such as attributional style or perceived control may be directly or indirectly linked to body dissatisfaction.[82]

WAYS TO IMPROVE THE RELATIONSHIP AMONG MEDIA USE, BODY IMAGE, AND EATING DISORDERS

A variety of intervention and prevention models designed to mitigate the influence of negative media messages on body image and eating behavior have been investigated, but most have shown limited success. A 2002 meta-analysis of prevention programs conducted in several industrialized countries found that programs that included media literacy and advocacy components were more successful than the other types of programs identified.[84] Media literacy and media education can be used to teach girls and women to become more active, critical consumers of appearance-related media to prevent the development of body dissatisfaction and disturbed eating behaviors. Media literacy interventions have been shown to decrease social comparison and internalization of the thin-ideal.[85] Additionally, exposure to healthy, normal-sized media figures can counteract negative messages. Viewing images of average-sized models has been shown to lower body-focused anxiety in women.[83,85]

However, short-term interventions may not be adequate to counteract the overall influence of predominant media messages. Because girls, especially, internalize negative attitudes about women's bodies at a young age, and because of the persistence of these internalized images despite counterimages, a complete shift away from the normative use of unrealistic-looking models and actors may be necessary to reform the internalized images of a healthy ideal body in the minds of the next generation of children and adolescents.[65] Some media campaigns, such as the Dove "Real Beauty" campaign, which uses real women in advertisements for beauty products, have proven successful for both advertisers and consumers.[86] Magazines such as *New Moon Girls*, which promote healthy body image and healthy active lifestyles for girls, have also been cited as examples of ways to counteract negative media messages.[79]

However, most media outlets are not motivated to move away from what they have found to be a successful paradigm. Advocates argue that because media will not self-regulate, it is necessary to implement policies and legislation designed to reduce or mitigate child and adolescent exposure to potentially harmful media messages.[87,88] This type of intervention, although it may ultimately be the most effective, is difficult to enact because of resistance from big media corporations. Any policy would have to balance the free-market interests of media corporations against the public health benefits. Despite some self-enforcement of content standards and government agency programming requirements, little top-down support exists for implementing or enforcing policies that would regulate or mandate media content.[87,88]

Popular with both parents and public health advocates, rating systems can function to alert audiences about potentially sensitive content while not interfering with the autonomy of media producers.[89] Movies, television, music, and video games all have some form of rating system, and these are usually based on age appropriateness and content. However, despite the popularity of the idea, actual rating systems as implemented are not effective because of inefficient implementation and lack of use.[89] Despite the challenges, advocates suggest the implementation of a two-pronged approach to content regulation. Policies that would restrict the portrayal of negative body images and eating attitudes and behaviors would include eliminating overly thin women or hypermuscular men. Concurrently, policies mandating the promotion of positive images would include healthy body sizes and healthy eating behaviors and attitudes.[79] Although no single intervention or prevention model has been completely successful, it is clear that vulnerability to body dissatisfaction and eating disorders in adolescence clearly occurs on multiple social fronts. For this reason, interventions that mitigate the effects of potentially harmful media messages must also occur at multiple social levels.

REFERENCES

1. Smolak L. Body image in children and adolescents: where do we go from here? Body Image 2004;1:15–28.
2. Ferrer-García M, Gutiérrez-Maldonado J. The use of virtual reality in the study, assessment, and treatment of body image in eating disorders and nonclinical samples: a review of the literature. Body Image 2012;9(1):1–11.
3. Maxwell MA, Cole DA. Development and initial validation of the adolescent responses to body dissatisfaction measure. Psychol Assess, in press.
4. McCabe MP, Ricciardelli LA, Finemore J. The role of puberty, media and popularity with peers on strategies to increase weight, decrease weight and increase muscle tone among adolescent boys and girls. J Psychosom Res 2002;52(3):145–53.
5. Siegel JM, Yancey AK, Aneshensel CS, et al. Body image, perceived pubertal timing, and adolescent mental health. J Adolesc Health 1999;25(2):155–65.
6. Dixit S, Agarwal G, Singh J, et al. A study on consciousness of adolescent girls about their body image. Indian J Community Med 2011;36(3):197–202.
7. Ferreiro F, Seoane G, Senra C. Gender-related risk and protective factors for depressive symptoms and disordered eating in adolescence: a 4-year longitudinal study. J Youth Adolesc, in press.
8. Gondoli DM, Corning AF, Salafia EH, et al. Heterosocial involvement, peer pressure for thinness, and body dissatisfaction among young adolescent girls. Body Image 2011;8(2):143–8.
9. Wojtowicz AE, von Ranson KM. Weighing in on risk factors for body dissatisfaction: a one-year prospective study of middle-adolescent girls. Body Image 2012;9(1):20–30.
10. Ricciardelli LA, McCabe MP, Holt KE, et al. A biopsychosocial model for understanding body image and body change strategies among children. J Appl Dev Psychol 2003;4(4):475–95.
11. Eshkevari E, Rieger E, Longo MR, et al. Increased plasticity of the bodily self in eating disorders. Psychol Med 2011;5:1–10.

12. Lethbridge J, Watson HJ, Egan SJ, et al. The role of perfectionism, dichotomous thinking, shape and weight overvaluation, and conditional goal setting in eating disorders. Eat Behav 2011;12(3):200–6.
13. Hudson JI, Hiripi E, Pope HG, et al. The prevalence and correlates of eating disorders in the National Comorbidity Survey Replication. Biol Psychiatry 2007; 61:348–58.
14. Hay PJ, Mond J, Buttner P, et al. Eating disorder behaviors are increasing: findings from two sequential community surveys in South Australia. PLoS One 2008; 3(2):e1541.
15. Swanson SA, Crow SJ, Le Grange D, et al. Prevalence and correlates of eating disorders in adolescents. Results from the national comorbidity survey replication adolescent supplement. Arch Gen Psychiatry 2011;68: 714–23.
16. Hoek HW. Incidence, prevalence and mortality of anorexia nervosa and other eating disorders. Curr Opin Psychiatry 2006;19:389–94.
17. Hoek HW, van Hoeken D. Review of the prevalence and incidence of eating disorders. Int J Eat Disord 2003;34:383–96.
18. Currin L, Schmidt U, Treasure J, et al. Time trends in eating disorder incidence. Br J Psychol 2005;186:132–5.
19. Nemeroff CJ, Stein RI, Diehl NS, et al. From the Cleavers to the Clintons: role choices and body orientation as reflected in magazine article content. Int J Eat Disord 1994;16:167–76.
20. Ballentine LW, Ogle JP. The making and unmaking of body problems in Seventeen Magazine. Fam Consum Sci Res J 2005;33(4):281–305.
21. Thompson-Brenner H, Boisseau CL, St. Paul MS. Representation of ideal figure size in ebony magazine: a content analysis. Body Image 2011;8:373–8.
22. Saucier JA, Caron SL. An investigation of content and media images in gay men's magazines. J Homosex 2008;55(3):504–23.
23. Milillo D. Sexuality sells: a content analysis of lesbian and heterosexual women's bodies in magazine advertisements. J Lesbian Stud 2008;12(4): 381–92.
24. Labre MP. Burn fat, build muscle: a content analysis of men's health and men's fitness. Int J Mens Health 2005;4(2):187–200.
25. Klein H, Shiffman KS. Messages about physical attractiveness in animated cartoons. Body Image 2006;3:353–63.
26. Northrup T, Liebler C. The good, the bad, and the beautiful: beauty ideals on the Disney & Nickelodeon channels. Paper presented at the International Communications Association Children, Adolescents, and the Media Interest Group. Singapore, 2008. Chicago (IL): May 25, 2009.
27. Robinson T, Callister M, Jankoski T. Portrayal of body weight on children's television sitcoms: a content analysis. Body Image 2008;5:141–51.
28. Fouts G, Burggraf K. Television situation comedies: female body images and verbal reinforcements. Sex Roles 1999;40(5–6):473–81.
29. White S, Brown NJ, Ginsburg SL. Diversity of body types in network television programming: a content analysis. Comm Res Reports 2010;16(4):386–92.
30. Fouts G, Vaughan K. Television situation comedies: male weight, negative references, and audience reactions. Sex Roles 2002;46(11/12):439–42.
31. Zhang Y, Dion TL, Conrad K. Female body image as a function of themes in rap music videos: a content analysis. 2010;62(11/12):787–97.
32. Herbozo S, Tantleff-Dunn S, Gokee-Larose J, et al. Beauty and thinness messages in children's media: a content analysis. Eat Disord 2004;12:21–34.

33. Alsip MK. Does evil have a shape? Comparing body types of heroes and villains in Disney animations. Paper presented at: Annual Meeting of the International Communication Association; Suntec City, Singapore; June 23, 2010.

34. Morrison TG, Halton M. Buff, tough, and rough: representations of muscularity in action motion pictures. J Mens Stud 2009;17(1):57–74.

35. Martins N, Williams DC, Harrison K, et al. A content analysis of female body imagery in video games. Sex Roles 2009;61:824–36.

36. Martins N, Williams DC, Ratan RA, et al. Virtual muscularity: a content analysis of male video game characters. Body Image 2011;8:43–51.

37. Hussin M, Frazier S, Thompson JK. Fat stigmatization on YouTube: a content analysis. Body Image 2011;8:90–2.

38. Borzekowski DLG, Schenk S, Wilson JL, et al. e-Ana and e-Mia: a content analysis of pro-eating disorder web sites. Am J Public Health 2010;100(8):1526–34.

39. Hancox RJ, Milne RJ, Poulton R. Association between child and adolescent television viewing and adult health: a longitudinal birth cohort study. Lancet 2004;364:257–62.

40. van den Berg P, Neumark-Sztainer D, Hannan PJ, et al. Is dieting advice from magazines helpful or harmful? Five-year associations with weight-control behaviors and psychological outcomes in adolescents. Pediatrics 2007;119(1):e30–7.

41. Martínez-González M, Gual P, Lahoriga F, et al. Parental factors, mass media influences, and the onset of eating disorders in a prospective population-based cohort. Pediatrics 2003;111(2):315–20.

42. Borzekowski DL, Robinson TN, Killen JD. Does the camera add ten pounds? Media use, perceived importance of appearance, and weight concerns among teenage girls. J Adolesc Health 2000;26:36–41.

43. Harrison K, Hefner V. Media exposure, current and future body ideals, and disordered eating among preadolescent girls: a longitudinal panel study. J Youth Adolesc 2006;35(2):146–56.

44. Harper K, Sperry S, Thompson JK. Viewership of pro-eating disorder websites: association with body image and eating disturbances. Int J Eat Disord 2008; 41:92–5.

45. Peebles R, Wilson JL, Borzekowski DL, et al. Disordered eating in a digital age: eating behaviors, health and quality of life in users of websites with pro-eating disorder content, in press.

46. Goodwin H, Haycraft E, Meyer C. Sociocultural correlates of compulsive exercise: is the environment important in fostering a compulsivity towards exercise among adolescents? Body Image 2011;8(4):390–5.

47. Elgin J, Pritchard M. Gender differences in disordered eating and its correlates. Eat Weight Disord 2006;11(3):e96–101.

48. Harrison K, Bond BJ. Gaming magazines and the drive for muscularity in preadolescent boys: a longitudinal examination. Body Image 2007;4:269–77.

49. Carper TL, Negy C, Tantleff-Dunn S. Relations among media influence, body image, eating concerns, and sexual orientation in men: a preliminary investigation. Body Image 2010;7(4):301–9.

50. Austin SB, Ziyadeh N, Kahn JA, et al. Sexual orientation, weight concerns, and eating-disordered behaviors in adolescent girls and boys. J Am Acad Child Adolesc Psychiatry 2004;43(9):1115–23.

51. Taveras EM, Rifas-Shiman SL, Field AE, et al. The influence of wanting to look like media figures on adolescent physical activity. J Adolesc Health 2004;35:41–50.

52. Young AF, Gabriel S, Sechrist GB. The skinny on celebrities: parasocial relationships moderate the effects of thin media figures on women's body image. Social Psych Pers Sc, in press. DOI:10.1177/1948550611434785.

53. Groesz LM, Levine MP, Murnen SK. The effect of experimental presentation of thin media images on body satisfaction: a meta-analytic review. Int J Eat Disord 2002; 31(1):1–16.

54. Hawkins N, Richards PS, Granley HM, et al. The impact of exposure to the thin-ideal media image on women. Eat Disord 2004;12(1):35–50.

55. Bardone-Cone AM, Cass KM. What does viewing a pro-anorexia website do? An experimental examination of website exposure and moderating effects. Int J Eat Disord 2007;40(6):537–48.

56. Jett S, LaPorte DJ, Wanchisn J. Impact of exposure to pro-eating disorder web-sites on eating behaviour in college women. Eur Eat Disord Rev 2010;18(5): 410–6.

57. Joshi R, Herman CP, Polivy J. Self-enhancing effects of exposure to thin-body images. Int J Eat Disord 2004;35(3):333–41.

58. Stice E, Spangler D, Agras WS. Exposure to media-portrayed thin-ideal images adversely affects vulnerable girls: a longitudinal experiment. J Soc Clin Psych 2001;20:270–88.

59. Legenbauer T, Rühl I, Vocks S. Influence of appearance-related TV commercials on body image state. Behav Modif 2008;32(3):352–71.

60. Chen H, Jackson T. Gender and age group differences in mass media and inter-personal influences on body dissatisfaction among Chinese adolescents. Sex Roles 2012;66:3–20.

61. Padgett J, Biro FM. Different shapes in different cultures: body dissatisfaction, overweight, and obesity in African-American and Caucasian females. J Pediatr Adolesc Gynecol 2003;16(6):349–54.

62. Presnell K, Bearman SK, Stice E. Risk factors for body dissatisfaction in adoles-cent boys and girls: a prospective study. Int J Eat Disord 2004;36(4):389–401.

63. López-Guimerà G, Levine MP, Sanchez-Carracedo D, et al. Influence of mass media on body image and eating disordered attitudes and behaviors in females: a review of effects and processes. Media Psychol 2010;13(4):387–416.

64. Bell BT, Dittmar H. Does media type matter? The role of identification in adoles-cent girls' media consumption and the impact of different thin-ideal media on body image. Sex Roles 2011;65(7/8):478–90.

65. Dittmar H, Halliwell E, Ive S. Does Barbie make girls want to be thin? The effect of experimental exposure to images of dolls on the body image of 5-to 8-year-old girls. Dev Psychol 2006;42(2):283–92.

66. Tiggemann M, Polivy J, Hargreaves D. The processing of thin ideals in fashion magazines: a source of social comparison or fantasy? J Soc Clin Psychol 2009;28(1):73–93.

67. Harrison K, Hefner V. Media exposure, current and future body ideals, and disordered eating among preadolescent girls. J Youth Adolesc 2006;35(2): 146–56.

68. Levine MP, Harrison K. Media's role in the perpetuation and prevention of nega-tive body image and disordered eating. In: Kevin J, editor. Handbook of eating disorders and obesity. Hoboken (NJ): John Wiley & Sons; 2004. p. 695–717.

69. Vartanian LR, Hopkinson MM. Social connectedness, conformity, and internaliza-tion of societal standards of attractiveness. Body Image 2010;7(1):86–9.

70. Hargreaves DA, Tiggemann M. Muscular ideal media images and men's body image: social comparison processing and individual vulnerability. Psychol Men Masc 2009;10(2):109–19.

71. Kennedy PF, Martin MC. Social comparison and the beauty of advertising models: the role of motives for comparison. Adv Consum Res 1994;21(1):365–71.

72. Cafri G, Yamamiya Y, Brannick M, et al. The Influence of Sociocultural Factors on Body Image: A Meta-Analysis. Clinical Psychology: Science and Practice 2005; 12(4):421–33.
73. Grabe S, Ward LM, Hyde JS. The role of the media in body image concerns among women: a meta-analysis of experimental and correlational studies. Psychol Bull 2008;134(3):460–76.
74. López-Guimerà G, Levine MP, Sanchez-Carracedo D, et al. Influence of mass media on body image and eating disordered attitudes and behaviors in females: a review of effects and processes. Media Psych 2010;13(4):387–416.
75. Dittmar H. How do "body perfect" ideals in the media have a negative impact on body image and behaviors? Factors and processes related to self and identity. J Soc Clin Psychol 2009;28(1):1–8.
76. Field AE, Camargo CA, Taylor CB, et al. Peer, parent, and media influences on the development of weight concerns and frequent dieting among preadolescent and adolescent girls and boys. Pediatrics 2001;107(1):54–60.
77. Turner HM, Rose KS, Cooper MJ. Parental bonding and eating disorder symptoms in adolescents: the mediating role of core beliefs. Eat Behav 2005;6(2): 113–8.
78. Stice E, Spangler D, Agras WS. Exposure to media-portrayed thin-ideal images adversely affects vulnerable girls: a longitudinal experiment. J Soc Clin Psychol 2001;20:270–88.
79. Borzekowski DL, Bayer AM. Body image and media use among adolescents. Adolesc Med Clin 2005;16(2):289–313.
80. Dohnt HK, Tiggemann M. Body image concerns in young girls: the role of peers and media prior to adolescence. J Youth Adolesc 2006;35(2):135–45.
81. Gunther AC, Bolt D, Borzekowski DL, et al. Presumed influence on peer norms: how mass media indirectly affect adolescent smoking. J Comm 2006;56(1): 52–68.
82. Lawler M, Nixon E. Body dissatisfaction among adolescent boys and girls: the effects of body mass, peer appearance culture and internalization of appearance ideals. J Youth Adolesc 2011;40(1):59–71.
83. Dittmar H, Halliwell E. Think "ideal" and feel bad? Using self-discrepancies to understand negative media effects. In: Dittmar H, Halliwell E, editors. Consumer culture, identity and well-being. New York: Psychology Press; 2008. p. 147–72.
84. Stice E. Risk and maintenance factors for eating pathology. Psychol Bull 2002; 128(5):825–48.
85. Halliwell E, Dittmar H, Dittmar H, et al. Does size matter? The impact of ultra-thin media models on women's body image and on advertising effectiveness. Consumer culture, identity, and well-being. 2008;121–46.
86. Johnston J, Taylor J. Feminist consumerism and fat activists: a comparative study of grassroots activism and the Dove Real Beauty campaign. Signs 2008;33(4): 941–66.
87. Boyce T. The media and obesity. Obes Rev 2007;8:201–5.
88. Kunkel D. Policy battles over defining children's educational television. Ann Am Acad Pol Soc Sci 1998;557(1):39–53.
89. Rideout V. Parents, media and public policy. In: Henry J, editor. A Kaiser Family Foundation survey. Washington, DC: Kaiser Family Foundation; 2004.

School Daze
Why are Teachers and Schools Missing the Boat on Media?

Victor C. Strasburger, MD

KEYWORDS

- Schools • Media • New technology • Sex education • Drug education

KEY POINTS

- Children and teens spend more time with media (>7 hours per day) than they do in school.
- Many schools are using new media (computer, the Internet, iPads, cell phones) in creative ways to keep students interested and motivated.
- Young people can have radically different learning styles, and new technology can be used to teach them differently.
- Sex education and drug education programs need to incorporate media and media literacy into their curricula.
- Given the immediacy of new technology (information at your fingertips 24/7), educators need to rethink some of the basic paradigms of education (eg, rote memorization).

[My doctor's] only gone to one medical school, but if you go online, you can get advice from all over the world.
        —Teenager quoted in TECHsex USA, 2011, p. 17[1]

...in a world where today's geography or social studies are quite literally tomorrow's history, it's intuitive that an easily updated, real-time text makes more sense than a 5-year-old, dog-eared and scribbled-on book that can be replaced only when there's sufficient funding.
        —Editorial, Albuquerque Journal, September 9, 2011[2]

There's a saying that the music is not in the piano and, in the same way, the learning is not in the device.
        —Professor Mark Warschauer, University of California, Irvine[3]

Department of Pediatrics, Division of Adolescent Medicine, University of New Mexico School of Medicine, MSC10 5590, 1 University of New Mexico School of Medicine, Albuquerque, NM 87131, USA
E-mail address: VStrasburger@salud.unm.edu

Pediatr Clin N Am 59 (2012) 705–715
doi:10.1016/j.pcl.2012.03.026   **pediatric.theclinics.com**

We need to build a more compelling narrative that digital literacy is no longer a luxury but a necessity.
—*S. Craig Watkins, author of the Young and the Digital: What the Migration to Social Network Sites, Games, and Anytime, Anywhere Media Means for Our Future[4]*

Most American schools are 50 years behind when it comes to using media wisely and incorporating new technology into the classroom.[5] Like medicine, the educational system has always been conservative and slow to adopt to new advances and new trends. As one author notes[6]:

The contemporary American classroom, with its grades and deference to the clock, is an inheritance from the late 19th century. During that period of titanic change, machines suddenly needed to run on time. Individual workers needed to willingly perform discrete operations as opposed to whole jobs. The industrial-era classroom, as a training ground for future factory workers, was retooled to teach tasks, obedience, hierarchy and schedules.

Unlike medicine, however, education only seems to have one yardstick with which to measure success: performance on standardized tests. As a result, new and creative approaches to teaching and learning fall by the wayside unless higher test scores can be documented.[7] This is a prescription for failure and is one of the reasons why American schools are so far behind in teaching students how to adapt to the brave new world of instant technology and connectedness. According to Cathy N. Davidson, codirector of the MacArthur Foundation Digital Media and Learning Competitions, 65% of today's grade-school students may end up doing jobs that have not even been invented yet.[6] Of course, funding schools in general and new technology specifically is a major hurdle for nearly all schools as well (**Fig. 1**).

MEDIA USE

Today's students spend more time with media than they do in school: between 7 and 11 hours per day, according to the 2010 Kaiser report.[8] The first "Internet class" (Class of 2015) is now just entering college (**Box 1**). Media are the leading leisure-time activity for children and adolescents, and they spend more time with media than they do in any other leisure-time activity other than sleeping.[9] By time criteria alone, one would think

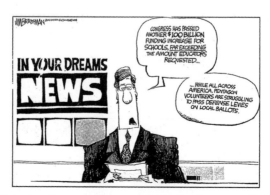

Fig. 1. (Copyright © Jim Borgman/Universal Press Syndicate. Used with permission of Universal Uclick.)

Box 1
The first "Internet class goes to college"

How the Class of 2015 Thinks Differently About Things

1. Amazon has never been just a river in South America.

2. Ferris Bueller and Sloane Peterson could be their parents.

3. They "swipe" cards, not merchandise.

4. "Don't touch that dial!"—what dial?

5. Video games have always had ratings.

6. Music has always been available via free downloads.

7. "PC" means Personal Computer, not Political Correctness.

8. Public schools have always made space available for advertising.

Adapted from McBride T, Nief R. The mindset list. Available at: http://themindsetlist.com/.

---

the media would be a force to be reckoned with; but the media also are powerful teachers of young people. Virtually every concern that teachers and parents have about children and teenagers is potentially influenced by the media: aggressive behavior,[10] sex,[11] drug use,[12] obesity,[13] eating disorders,[14] and depression.[15] Several studies have found a deterioration in academic performance with increasing screen time[16–22] and have linked increased screen time at a young age with the development of attention-deficit disorder and attention-deficit/hyperactivity disorder.[23–25] A recent longitudinal Canadian study of 1314 children at 29 months of age and in fourth grade found that for every additional hour of television viewed per day at 29 months of age, there was a 6% to 7% decrease in classroom participation, a 10% increase in victimization by classmates, a 9% decrease in physical activity, and a 5% increase in body mass index by the fourth grade.[26]

But the term "media" now means far more than television, movies, or music. "New" technology has become increasingly important as well, although there are only a few behavioral studies available to date. Nearly 90% of 8- to 18-year-olds now have Internet access at home, and one-third have access in their bedroom.[8] Half of young people surveyed say that they have a video game player in their room.[8] Both the Nielsen Company and the Pew Foundation have been tracking new media use:[27,28]

- American 18-year-olds now average nearly 40 hours per week online from their home computers, including 5.5 hours of streaming video.
- Nearly all teenagers (93%) now use the Internet. In a 2009 survey, 70% of 12- to 17-year-olds owned a cell phone, and 80% owned an iPod and a game console.
- More than 78% of 12- to 17-year-olds have visited social networks or read blogs.
- Some 75% of 12- to 17-year-olds now own cell phones, up from 45% in 2004. Nearly all teens (88%) are texters.
- Virtually all teenagers now have MP3 players, and they often use high-volume settings.[29] The same goes for multitasking: nearly 40% of 7th to 12th graders say that they multitask frequently, listening to music (43%), using the computer (40%), or watching television (39%).[8] Some neuroscientists worry about how efficient multitasking really is and about its impact on the developing adolescent brain.[30]

MEDIA USE, SLEEP, AND SCHOOLS

Surprisingly, new research shows that teenagers need more sleep than older children do: 8 to 9 hours per night.[31,32] Yet media use is associated with less sleep, especially when so many different forms of media are now present in the bedroom.[8,33] Sleep deprivation has been associated with fatigue, neurocognitive impairment, increased risk of accidents, and poorer school performance.[33,34] Given the normal sleep pattern of most teenagers (staying up late at night and wanting to sleep late in the morning), does it make sense to start high-school classes earlier than grade-school or middle-school classes? School systems such as in Minneapolis have experimented with later starting times (as late as 9:00–9:30 AM), and have found significant improvements in classroom performance and test scores.[33–35]

HEALTH EDUCATION

Although most schools and school systems now have drug prevention and sex education programs, relatively few have kept pace with modern media and deal with media content (**Table 1**). Nationwide, 70% of schools still use Drug Abuse Resistance Education (DARE), even though multiple studies show that it is ineffective.[36,37] Part of its ineffectiveness is the absence of media education in the curriculum, for example, the impact of cigarette and alcohol advertising and depictions of drug use in movies and on television.[38] Similarly, sex education programs routinely ignore topics such as sex in the media and the absence of contraceptive advertising in American society.[39] Media can be part of the solution, not just part of the problem. Using media to educate children and teens about sex puts the subjects on kids' "home turf" and also helps them resist unhealthy media messages—one of the aims of media education.[40] The latter is absolutely crucial in the twenty-first century, yet the United States lags far behind other Western countries such as Canada, Australia, and the United Kingdom in incorporating media education into the everyday curriculum.[40] Numerous studies have now shown media education to be effective in preventing aggressive behavior,[41] drug use,[37,42,43] and even inappropriate sexual displays on social networking sites.[44] It is true that schools represent the final common denominator in society and therefore seem to have the ultimate responsibility for remedying all childhood ills. Nevertheless, teaching children about media can accomplish many useful health goals.[40]

USING NEW TECHNOLOGY IN THE CLASSROOM

Forty years ago, classroom teachers complained about the fast pace of the new children's show "Sesame Street," saying that it increased pressure on them to be

Table 1
What exactly are students taught about media?

	Grade School (%)	Middle School (%)	High School (%)
Students are taught the influence of media on (N = 1000 schools):			
Physical activity	43	53	63
Alcohol/drug use	51	78	89
Tobacco use	52	75	86
Sexual behavior	12	60	77
Violent behaviors	57	52	70

Data from Kann L, Telljohann SK, Wooley SF. Health education: results from the school health policies and programs study 2006. J School Health 2007;77(8):408–34.

entertainers so that their students' attention would not wander.[45] But the flip-side of the equation is that new technology in the classroom offers nearly limitless educational possibilities:

- More than 600 school districts are now using iPads instead of textbooks. iPads cost $500 to $600, but administrators at Brookfield High School in Connecticut estimate that they spend at least that much annually on every student's text-books, which does not include all of the add-ons (graphing calculators, dictio-naries, and so forth) available on the iPads.[3]
- A Los Angeles eighth-grade teacher has his students use Twitter to chime in with questions and answers during his presentations.[46] Similarly, Purdue University developed its own backchannel system, Hot Seat, which lets students post comments and questions online during lectures. It allows quiet or shy students to speak up.[7]
- A Spanish teacher in Wesley Chapel, Florida insists that her students bring their cell phones to class; she texts them in Spanish and they respond.[47]
- With a program called MealpayPlus, parents in more than 250 school districts can track their children's lunch purchases and see exactly what they are eating.[48] Many parents use an Internet program called iParent to track their children's attendance, school assignments, and performance. In Royal Oaks Schools in Michigan, parent-teacher conferences are conducted online.
- Many schools are experimenting with "blended learning": a shift to an online envi-ronment for at least part of the school day to improve learning and productivity.
- Special-education students may especially benefit from new technology.[49] At Westmark School in Encino, California, special-education students learn frac-tions via brightly colored, jungle-themed pie charts, they can ask their iPads how to spell and define words, and they can practice cursive writing via a tracing application.
- Teacher training is changing as well.[50] At the Teachers College of San Joaquin in Stockton, California, "multiple learning pathways" are emphasized: that is, the need to approach subjects from many different angles to accommodate different learning styles. At Cal State—Fullerton, student teachers are immersed in inter-active whiteboards, digital media tools, and Web 2.0 teaching strategies. At the University of Central Florida, teaching apprenticeships are done virtually.
- At the cutting edge of new technology, avatars are being used to interact with grade-school students one on one. Avatars can be customized for each individual, follow their eye-tracking on the computer screen, and keep them motivated.[51]

PROBLEMS WITH NEW TECHNOLOGY

With any new technology come new problems. Students may be physically present in the classroom, but downloading videos online or texting classmates. New technology has also brought new issues and concerns into schools. Should students be allowed to carry cell phones? Should they be linked up to the Internet in class? If computers are used in class, what kind of screening or blocking mechanism is appropriate? Should school libraries use Internet blocking technology? Should students be allowed to complete joint projects in chat rooms online? How should schools deal with the prob-lems of Internet bullying and harassment or sexting (sending sexually explicit pictures via cell phone) (**Table 2**)? According to 2 separate studies, 10% to 33% of teenagers have experienced online bullying or harassment,[52,53] and as many as 20% of

Table 2
Are cybersafety and cyberethics being taught in schools? Zogby/463 survey of 1012 teachers and 402 school administrators in February 2011

Does your school do a good job preparing students re: cybersafety and cyberethics?

	Yes (%)	No (%)	Not sure (%)
Teachers	51	41	4
Administrators	81	16	2

How prepared are you to talk about cyberbullying?

	Not Prepared (%)	Prepared (%)	Not sure (%)
Teachers	18	54	1
Administrators	12	63	2

How prepared are you to talk about sexting?

	Not Prepared (%)	Prepared (%)	Not sure (%)
Teachers	20	58	3
Administrators	13	69	23

Yet, in the past 12 months before being surveyed, less than one-third of teachers taught students about:

Online content that scares them
"Netiquette"
Hate speech
Risks of social networking sites
Cyberbullying
Sexting

In the past 12 months, 36% of teachers spent 0 hours on training on these topics within their school districts. Another 40% spent <3 hours

Data from National Cyber Security Alliance, Microsoft Corporation, Zogby/463. The state of K-12 cyberethics, cybersafety and cybersecuirty curriculum in the United States. 2011. Available at: StaySafeOnline.org. Accessed September 21, 2011.

teenagers have engaged in sexting,[54] although the actual prevalence is probably closer to 5% according to the most recent study.[55]

IS THERE A NEED FOR A NEW EDUCATIONAL PARADIGM?

Arguably, new technology should be revolutionizing fundamental educational strategies. Some might question why we ask students to memorize dozens of names and dates in United States history when in the near future, their wristwatches and cell phones will be 10-gigabyte computers capable of instantaneously spitting out whatever facts are needed (**Fig. 2**). Instead, the need to teach critical thinking and how to sift through the vast amount of information—some of it good, some of it not so good—in written materials, on television, and on the Internet has become of paramount importance.

Different learning styles can now be accommodated using different technologies, but the fundamentals of reading and writing do not necessarily need to be discarded simply because of digital and visual media. Numerous reading apps support word recognition and fluency. More specialized programs such as Highlighter enable students to practice reading comprehension tactics.[56] For writing, one of the basic premises of Web 2.0 is collaboration and peer input, and file sharing allows students to do exactly that. Programs such as Google Docs give teachers options for writing

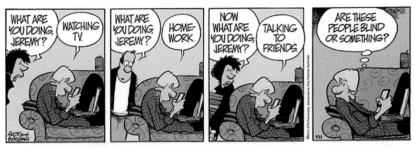

Fig. 2. (ZITS © ZITS PATNERSHIP, KING FEATURES SYNDICATE. Used with permission.)

exercises that are not confined to a single 50-minute class period.[56] Similarly, the availability of new technology should be making classroom teaching easier and more effective. Textbooks remain important, but there are instances whereby a video (eg, Ken Burn's extraordinary *Civil War* series) might be used to augment a textbook. Teachers can now choose from 10 different DVD versions of *Romeo and Juliet* (and Shakespeare wrote his plays to be performed and seen, not to be read),[5] so it makes little sense to torture middle-school students with trying to understand and master Elizabethan English.

COMMERCIALISM AND SCHOOLS

In the past 2 decades, advertisers have specifically targeted school populations to reach younger and younger audiences, and many cash-strapped schools have cooperated.[57] Advertisers have specifically targeted younger and younger children in classrooms.[57] Channel One, which is 10 minutes of current-events programming along with 2 minutes of commercials, continues to be seen in 8000 middle and high schools around the country.[58] It is seen by 40% of American teenagers.[57] Junk food ads are ubiquitous, and violent movies and prescription drugs are advertised.[59] Structured educational materials are free curricula produced by major corporations and include such items as a Campbell's soup "Prego Thickness Experiment," comparing the thickness of Prego and Ragu spaghetti sauces, and materials by Chevron challenging the existence of global warming.[57] In 2006, book fairs generated $404 million for the publisher Scholastic, which then sells noneducational products for major companies such as Disney and Nickelodeon.[60]

SUMMARY

Solutions will not be easy. Schools and teachers will not like or appreciate outsiders trying to help with educational policy. Pediatricians, however, are also media experts, and media are now inextricably linked with schools and learning. Possible solutions now include:

- Later starting times, especially for high schoolers
- Incorporating media-related elements into sex education and drug prevention programs
- Teaching media education in a K-12 fashion, including the proper use and "etiquette" of new technology
- Helping teachers use new technologies in the classroom
- Formulating school rules about cell phone use, texting, sexting, and cyberbullying

- Banning advertisers and advertising from school
- Formulating a new definition of what it means to be "educated," and jettisoning the need for rote memorization (except for, perhaps, the multiplication tables in grade school).

Schools, and the American education system, must change. The only question is how long will it take before the traditionally conservative educational system catches up with rapidly advancing new technology? Until then, the American educational system will remain decades behind the times and hopelessly out of date.

REFERENCES

1. Boyar R, Levine D, Zensius N. TECHsex USA: youth sexuality and reproductive health in the digital age. Oakland (CA): ISIS, Inc; 2011.
2. You may never have to crack a book again [editorial]. Albuquerque Journal 2011;A6. Available at: http://www.abqjournal.com/main/2011/09/09/opinion/you-may-never-have-to-crack-a-book-again.html. Accessed March 16, 2012.
3. Reitz S. Many US schools adding iPads, trimming textbooks. Associated Press; 2011. Available at: http://www.msnbc.msn.com/id/44384057/ns/technology_and_science-tech_and_gadgets/t/many-us-schools-adding-ipads-trimming-textbooks/. Accessed September 26, 2011.
4. Barseghian T. For at-risk youth, is learning digital media a luxury. MindShift; 2011. Available at: http://www.pbs.org/mediashift/2011/07/is-digital-education-a-luxury-for-at-risk-youth209.html. Accessed September 26, 2011.
5. Strasburger VC. Why are teachers and schools so clueless about the media? Hampton (IA): Liberal Opinion Week; 2010. p. 24.
6. Heffernan V. Education needs a digital-age upgrade. New York Times; 2011. Available at: http://opinionator.blogs.nytimes.com/2011/08/07/education-needs-a-digital-age-upgrade/. Accessed September 26, 2011.
7. Gabriel T, Richtel M. Inflating the software report card. New York Times; 2011. Available at: http://www.nytimes.com/2011/10/09/technology/a-classroom-software-boom-but-mixed-results-despite-the-hype.html?pagewanted=all. Accessed March 28, 2012.
8. Rideout V. Generation M2: media in the lives of 8- to 18-year-olds. Menlo Park (CA): Kaiser Family Foundation; 2010.
9. Strasburger VC, Jordan AB, Donnerstein E. Health effects of media on children and adolescents. Pediatrics 2010;125:756–67.
10. Strasburger VC, AAP Council on Communications and Media. Media violence (policy statement). Pediatrics 2009;124:1495–503.
11. Strasburger VC, AAP Council on Communications and Media. Adolescent sexuality and the media (policy statement). Pediatrics 2010;126(3):576–82.
12. Strasburger VC, AAP Council on Communications and Media. Adolescents, substance use, and the media (policy statement). Pediatrics 2010;126(4):791–9.
13. Strasburger VC, AAP Council on Communications and Media. Children, adolescents, obesity, and the media. Pediatrics 2011;128:201–8.
14. Jordan A, Kramer-Golinkoff E, Strasburger V. Do the media cause obesity & eating disorders? Adolesc Med State Art Rev 2008;19:431–49.
15. Primack BA, Swanier B, Georgiopoulos AM, et al. Association between media use in adolescence and depression in young adulthood: a longitudinal study. Arch Gen Psychiatry 2009;66:181–8.

16. Hancox RJ, Milne BJ, Poultn R. Association of television viewing during childhood with poor educational achievement. Arch Pediatr Adolesc Med 2005;159(7): 614–8.

17. Zimmerman FJ, Christakis DA. Children's television viewing and cognitive outcomes: a longitudinal analysis of national data. Arch Pediatr Adolesc Med 2005;159(7):619–25.

18. Borzekowski DL, Robinson TN. The remote, the mouse, and the No. 2 pencil: the household media environment and academic achievement among third grade students. Arch Pediatr Adolesc Med 2005;159(7):607–13.

19. Sharif I, Sargent JD. Association between television, movie, and video game exposure and school performance. Pediatrics 2006;118:e1061–70.

20. Sharif I, Wills TA, Sargent JA. Effect of visual media use on school performance: a prospective study. J Adolesc Health 2010;46:52–61.

21. Weis R, Cerankosky BC. Effects of video-game ownership on young boys' academic and behavioral functioning: a randomized, controlled study. Psychol Sci 2010. Available at: http://pss.sagepub.com/content/early/2010/02/17/0956797610362670. abstract. Accessed September 3, 2011.

22. Mossle T, Leimann M, Rehbein F, et al. Media use and school achievement—boys at risk? Br J Dev Psychol 2010;38(Pt 3):699–725.

23. Christakis DA, Zimmerman FJ, DiGiuseppe DL, et al. Early television exposure and subsequent attentional problems in children. Pediatrics 2004;113(4):708–13.

24. Swing EL, Gentile DA, Anderson CA, et al. Television and video game exposure and the development of attention problems. Pediatrics 2010;126:214–21.

25. Lillard AS, Peterson J. The immediate impact of different types of television on young children's executive function. Pediatrics 2011;128:644–9.

26. Pagani LS, Fitzpatrick C, Barnett TA, et al. Prospective associations between early childhood television exposure and academic, psychosocial, and physical well-being by middle childhood. Arch Pediatr Adolesc Med 2010;164:425–31.

27. Nielsen Company. State of the media: TV usage trends: Q3 and Q4 2010. New York: Nielsen Company; 2011.

28. Lenhart A. Teens and sexting. Washington, DC: Pew Internet & American Life Project; 2009. Available at: http://www.pewinternet.org/~/media//Files/Reports/2009/PIP_Teens_and_Sexting.pdf. Accessed October 26, 2011.

29. Vogel I, Vershuure H, van der Ploeg CP, et al. Adolescents and MP3 players: too many risks, too few precautions. Pediatrics 2009;123:e953–8.

30. Small G, Vorgan G. iBrain: surviving the technology alteration of the modern mind. New York: Harper Collins; 2008.

31. Millman RP, Working Group on Sleepiness in Adolescents/Young Adults, American Academy of Pediatrics, Committee on Adolescence. Technical report: excessive sleepiness in adolescents and young adults: causes, consequences, and treatment strategies. Pediatrics 2005;115(6):1774–86.

32. Sass AE, Kaplan DW. Sleep and sleep disorders in adolescents. Adolesc Med State Art Rev 2010;21(3):401–560.

33. Zimmerman FJ. Children's media use and sleep problems: issues and unanswered questions. Menlo Park (CA): Kaiser Family Foundation; 2008.

34. McKnight-Eily LR, Eaton DK, Lowry R, et al. Relationships between hours of sleep and health-risk behaviors in US adolescent students. Prev Med 2011;53(4/5):271–3.

35. Wahlstrom K. School start time and sleepy teens. Arch Pediatr Adolesc Med 2010;164:676–7.

36. West SL, O'Neal KK. Prject D.A.R.E. outcome effectiveness revisited. Am J Public Health 2004;94:1027–9.

37. Botvin GJ, Griffin KW. Models of prevention: School - based programs. In: Lowinson JH, Ruiz P, Millman RB, et al, editors. Substance abuse: a comprehensive textbook. 4th edition. Philadelphia: Lippincott, Williams & Wilkins; 2005. p. 1211–29.

38. Strasburger VC. Children, adolescents, drugs, and the media. In: Singer DG, Singer JL, editors. Handbook of children and the media. Thousand Oaks (CA): Sage; 2012. p. 419–54.

39. Strasburger VC. Adolescents, sex, and the media. Adolesc Med State Art Rev 2012;23(1):15–33.

40. Strasburger VC, Hogan MJ, AAP Council on Communications and Media. Media education (policy statement). Pediatrics 2010;126:1012–7.

41. Rosenkoetter LI, Rosenkoetter SE, Acock AC. Television violence: an intervention to reduce its impact on children. J Appl Dev Psychol 2009;30(4): 361–97.

42. Primack BA, Fine D, Yang CK, et al. Adolescents' impressions of antismoking media literacy education: qualitative results from a randomized controlled trial. Health Educ Res 2009;24(4):608–21.

43. Austin EW, Johnson KK. Effects of general and alcohol-specific media literacy training on children's decision making about alcohol. J Health Commun 1997;2(1): 17–42.

44. Moreno MA, VanderStoep A, Parks MR, et al. Reducing at-risk adolescents' display of risk behavior on a social networking web site. Arch Pediatr Adolesc Med 2009;163(1):35–41.

45. Garner R. We can't compete with television, teachers complain. The Independent; 2009. Available at: http://www.independent.co.uk/news/education/education-news/we-cant-compete-with-television-teachers-complain-1668264.html. Accessed October 24, 2011.

46. Simon D. Twitter finds a place in the classroom. CNN.com; 2011. Available at: http://articles.cnn.com/2011-06-08/tech/twitter.school_1_twitter-students-classroom discussions?_s=PM: TECH. Accessed October 31, 2011.

47. O'Meara C. Teachers begin using cell phones for class lessons. Associated Press; 2009. Available at: http://www.syracuse.com/news/index.ssf/2009/11/teachers_begin_using_cell_phon.html. Accessed October 31, 2011.

48. Samuels A. Parents go online to see where the lunch money goes. L.A. Times; 2008. Available at: http://latimesblogs.latimes.com/technology/2008/08/parents-go-onli.html. Accessed October 31, 2011.

49. Rosenblum L. Change the future of special education? There's an app for that. 2011. Available at: http://encino.patch.com/articles/change-the-future-of-special-education-theres-an-app-for-that. Accessed October 31, 2011.

50. Bernard S. Five progressive schools of education. Mindshift.kqed.org; 2010. Available at: http://mindshift.kqed.org/2011/06/five-progressive-schools-of-education/. Accessed October 31, 2011.

51. Taylor E. 10 amazing ways avatars are being used in education. Available at: http://www.accreditedonlinecolleges.com/blog/2010/10-amazing-ways-avatars-are-being-used-in-education/. Accessed November 2, 2011.

52. Williams KR, Guerra NG. Prevalence and predictors of Internet bullying. J Adolesc Health 2007;41:S14–21.

53. Ybarra ML, Mitchell KJ. How risky are social networking sites? A comparison of places online where youth sexual solicitation and harassment occurs. Pediatrics 2008;121:e350–7.

54. National Campaign to Prevent Teen and Unplanned Pregnancy. Sex and tech. Washington, DC: National Campaign to Prevent Teen and Unplanned Pregnancy; 2008.

55. Mitchell K, Finkelhor D, Jones L, et al. Prevalence and characteristics of youth sexting: a national study. Pediatrics 2012;129:1–8.

56. Nolan S. How technology fuels learning. 2011. Available at: http://mindshift.kqed.org/2011/09/how-technology-fuels-learning/. Accessed October 31, 2011.

57. Kanner AD. Today's class brought to you by...Tikkun Magazine, January/February, 2008. p. 24–5. Available at: http://www.commercialfreechildhood.org/articles/featured/todaysclass.pdf. Accessed October 31, 2011.

58. Available at: http://www.channelone.com/about/faq/. Accessed October 31, 2011.

59. Campaign for a Commercial-Free Childhood. Advocates to Channel One: stop marketing prescription drugs to children [press release]. 2008. Available at: http://commercialfreechildhood.org/pressreleases.channelonedrugs.htm. Accessed October 31, 2011.

60. Campaign for a Commercial-Free Childhood. Putting the book back in book fair. 2007. Available at: http://commercialfreechildhood.org/articles/featured/puttingthe.htm. Accessed October 31, 2011.

Ten Years of TeenHealthFX.com
A Case Study of an Adolescent Health Web Site

Dina L.G. Borzekowski, EdD[a],*, Cathy McCarthy, MPH[b],
Walter D. Rosenfeld, MD[c]

KEYWORDS

- Adolescents • Internet • Online health information • Web sites

KEY POINTS

- Reasons for going online include communication and entertainment, but adolescent users also turn to this resource for health information.
- Health Web sites can offer youth a way to easily access sensitive health information, explore topics anonymously, and receive direct, candid answers from health professionals.
- TeenHealthFX is a health information Web site that was created in 1999 by the Atlantic Health System Goryeb Children's Hospital, Morristown Medical Center, and Overlook Medical Center.
- Although funding and maintenance of such a Web site can be substantial, the rewards to the young people who use it, the professionals who operate it, and the community that it serves are great.
- Those considering development of a technology-based intervention to reach young people can learn from the case history of TeenHealthFX.

More so than any other age group, adolescents and young adults are early adopters of emerging technology. Most (93%) US teenagers ages 12 to 17 are online and 80% of these youth have broadband access from their homes.[1] Reasons for going online include communication and entertainment, but young users also turn to this resource for health information.[1,2] Internationally, the Internet is a popular tool to find sensitive information, especially on topics such as sex, weight loss, and risky behaviors.[3,4]

Although there are concerns in using emerging technology for health information and behavioral advice,[5–7] the Internet, in contrast to in-person interactions with health providers, allows ease of access in an anonymous and nonpunitive way.[3,4,8] Across

The authors have indicated that they have no financial relationships relevant to this article to disclose.
[a] Department of Health, Behavior and Society, Johns Hopkins Bloomberg School of Public Health, 624 North Broadway, #745, Baltimore, MD 21205, USA; [b] Morristown Medical Center, Atlantic Health System, Morristown, NJ 07960, USA; [c] Goryeb Children's Hospital, Atlantic Health System, Morristown, NJ 07960, USA
* Corresponding author.
E-mail address: dborzeko@jhsph.edu

Pediatr Clin N Am 59 (2012) 717–727
doi:10.1016/j.pcl.2012.03.018
0031-3955/12/$ – see front matter © 2012 Elsevier Inc. All rights reserved.
pediatric.theclinics.com

generations, adolescents have sought honest, direct answers to important but embarrassing questions about health; emerging technologies provide a much-needed venue to obtain relevant information without geographic, time, financial, and personal barriers.

This article is a case study, offering the story of TeenHealthFX. From discussion of this specific Web site, those interested in how youth access online health information can learn of the positive and negative aspects of delivering health messages through the Internet. Beyond describing the process involved in creating and maintaining TeenHealthFX, this article discusses the challenges of providing online health information to adolescents via new technology.

TEENHEALTHFX's BEGINNING

TeenHealthFX is a project of the Atlantic Health System Goryeb Children's Hospital, Morristown Medical Center, and Overlook Medical Center. The planning for this hospital–community collaborative initiative began in 1998 and was created with the assistance, advice, and support from the Morristown Health Department, County College of Morris, Morris School District, Child and Family Resources, New Jersey Department of Education, Morristown Medical Center Advisory Board, Community Health Department, and the Adolescent/Young Adult Center for Health at the Atlantic Health System's Goryeb Children's Hospital.

Every 3 years, community and board members of the Morristown Medical Center convene to establish their goals, driven by a community needs assessment. In 1998, this assessment revealed that adolescents lacked easy access to good and reliable health information. Despite a local and comprehensive adolescent medicine program, only a small proportion of local youth were having their health information concerns addressed. Given that most local youth were not accessing care and the emerging must-have status of the Internet, the community proposed that a Web site for adolescents and young adults be created. In early 1999, the Atlantic Health System Community Health Committee made up of Morris County community leaders and hospital employees gave $67,500 to initiate this effort.

TeenHealthFX's stated mission is to provide adolescent Internet users with an online resource for general and specific questions about physical and emotional health. As conceived, the Web site was also a tool to improve young people's health literacy and train them to navigate a challenging health care system. Additionally, the Web site was to assist youth living in the region (Northern New Jersey) with information about how to obtain local medical, mental health, and support services. An underlying goal of TeenHealthFX was and is to empower adolescents to improve their health through individual responsibility.

It is common for adolescents to believe that their health questions, behaviors, and physical changes are abnormal and even bizarre.[9] Because youth may be too embarrassed to seek important health care and advice,[10] resources must be confidential. Although candid, direct, and factual information is valued, it may not be readily available to young people through local services, many of which are already overburdened. Additionally, youth benefit from learning that what they consider a "unique" question or problem is also asked and/or faced by others. Although a Web site neither cannot nor should not replace one-on-one clinical advice, the developers of TeenHealthFX thought that it could serve as an ideal starting place to deliver essential, albeit sometimes uncomfortable, information.

ORIGINAL DESIGN AND MODIFICATIONS

After receiving initial funding, a coordinator was hired and a design committee was formed. Although resourceful and enthusiastic, those involved, like others joining the dot-com surge of the late 1990s, had limited direct experience in Web site design or management. The initial team consisted of the coordinator, adolescent medicine professionals, community leaders, and, most importantly, teenagers who also served on the newly formed Teen Advisory Committee (TAC). An outside Web site development firm was contracted to create the Web site. It took approximately 6 months to craft the Web site's first version.

TeenHealthFX went live in September 1999. **Fig. 1** presents an image of the first home page. The launch occurred at a neighborhood high school and local television news stations and newspapers featured stories about the Web site.

Without drawing on a specific communication theory, the design incorporated a user-friendly approach consistently involving static components of information and navigation bars on the page's top and left sides. Dynamic text or images appeared center right on the page (where the picture of the Wizard is on the home page). The top navigation bar included the TeenHealthFX logo, which was a link back to the home page. Below the TeenHealthFX logo, users could access the Emergency Help Now!, Links, About Us, Ask FX, and Rate Us sections using navigation buttons, and these buttons appeared throughout the Web site. The side toolbar featured navigation buttons for different subject categories. The original Web site's sections included

Ask FX: An area where visitors could post questions any time they wished to.

FX Answers: An area where visitors could find previously posted questions and answers. Visitors could search through categorized subject areas.

FX Links: A section that linked visitors to Web sites not associated with Morristown Medical Center but deemed by the research team and other health educators good medical and health resources. (External links are added to TeenHealthFX.com regularly in the Links section and in most of the questions in the FX Answers section of the site. Before any external links are included

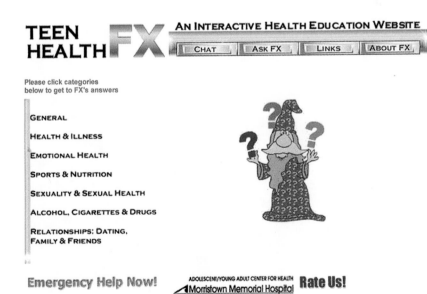

Fig. 1. The original TeenHealthFX home page, as it appeared in its released form in September 1999. (*Courtesy of* the Atlantic Health System; with permission.)

on the site, a trained educator thoroughly reviews them for relevance to the current question/answer or section of TeenHealthFX, accuracy of information in a teen-friendly format, good reputation of site authors, and that the external link is consistent with the philosophy of TeenHealthFX. In June 2006, the links on TeenHealthFX were re-reviewed and revised with several additions and deletions.)

Chat: A chat room moderated by medical professionals and health educators. This feature was canceled in May 2002, primarily because it was labor intensive and not cost efficient.

Emergency Help Now: A section that provided visitors with phone numbers for immediate medical and mental health services. Additionally, this section was a disclaimer page stating that TeenHealthFX was neither a crisis intervention Web site nor a substitute for medical care.

Despite growing use and appreciation, a common criticism was that the initial design was too juvenile. Focus groups and Web site surveys offered information from adolescents, who perceived TeenHealthFX's information as relevant and helpful but thought that the overall look was childish and colors used (gray and white) were corporate and plain looking. Responding to these concerns, a revision was done in conjunction with the design committee and a new Web site development company.

A redesigned TeenHealthFX was launched in September 2000 (**Fig. 2**). This Web site used bright colors (yellows, blues, and pinks) on a darkened (black and navy blue mix) background. Throughout the redesigned site, photographs of adolescents were featured. New sections were added, including

Teen Tips: A section created by the TAC that offered articles, tips, and feedback on common issues of concern to teenagers; some topics were mundane (eg, 9 Ways to Speed Up your Morning Ritual), whereas others were serious (eg, how to deal with traumatic events).

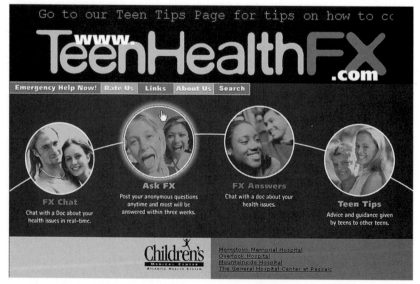

Fig. 2. The redesigned TeenHealthFX home page, as it appeared in its released form in September 2000. (*Courtesy of* the Atlantic Health System; with permission.)

SearchFX: An internal search using a keyword search to find relevant pages within the Web site.

The SearchFX feature was added for two reasons. First, it aided visitors in their search for answers to commonly asked questions. Second, it reduced the burden on the TeenHealthFX staff; it became impractical to answer every submitted question. Adolescents would be both reassured to see that they were not alone with their concerns as well as pleased to find immediate answers. The highlighted search engine button on the home page encouraged visitors to search first before submitting questions.

In late 2003, the Atlantic Health System had an external agency audit TeenHealthFX, with the primary goal of uncovering ways to increase traffic flow not only to Teen-HealthFX but also to the hospital's home page. This audit prompted another redesign. An established Web design and marketing firm (which was becoming easier to find) created the current version of TeenHealthFX. This version, which features a newspaper look with bright colors (orange and greens) and more photographs of real adolescents, went live in April 2004 (**Fig. 3**). In addition to the sections found in previous designs, the revised TeenHealthFX added the following sections:

Facts: Quick and easy to understand health facts. New facts appear each time a visitor logs on.
Hot Topics: A short paragraph, written by the TeenHealthFX professional staff, on current subjects, modified monthly.
Happenings: A page and links referencing local community programs and opportunities, available through the Atlantic Health System.
Quizzes: A short multiple-choice quiz on a relevant health subject. Approximately 7 different quizzes are cycled, so that visitors may view new quizzes each time

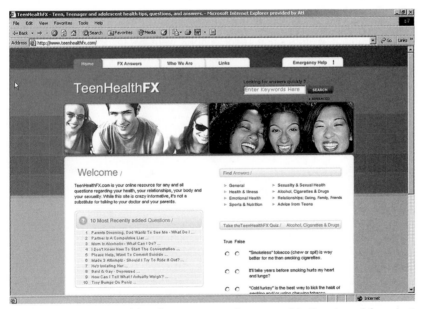

Fig. 3. The current TeenHealthFX home page, as it appeared in its released form in April 2004. (*Courtesy of* the Atlantic Health System; with permission.)

they visit the home page. Correct responses are available once a visitor completes the quiz.

Resource of the Month: Added in 2007, this section reviews books and other Web sites for adolescents.

Where Do You Stand: In 2007–2009, current and controversial issues were posted and adolescents encouraged to contribute their thoughts and feelings.

COSTS

Fig. 4 presents the annual cost for TeenHealthFX from 1999 through the end of 2009. The increase in 2002 reflects the costs involved in a major redesign, which included a search engine registration and using metatags to allow search engines, such as Google and Yahoo, to scan each Web site. The most significant ongoing cost for the site is supporting the salaries of the health educators involved. Through efficiencies developed and re-engineering of the site (described previously), this cost has been reduced but remains a factor. As from the beginning of its establishment, the leadership of the Atlantic Health System considers the operation of the site as providing a direct and unique benefit to the community. This is a good fit for a not-for-profit academic institution that includes in its mission improving the health status of the community.

WEB SITE USE

The anonymous nature of this Web site prevents collection of demographic data on previous and current users, including information on gender, age, and geographic residence. Unlike many health and youth Web sites, visitors do not register when they enter TeenHealthFX. Furthermore, TeenHealthFX does not use cookies, which is a text file sent by a server to a Web browser that authenticates, tracks, and maintains user-specific information.

Data on the Web site's traffic, however, are available. **Fig. 4** presents the annual numbers for unique visitors since TeenHealthFX went live in 1999. Considering data from 2000, the monthly average of unique visitors was 1818 and visitor sessions was 5864. In 2005, the monthly averages increased to around one hundred times the amount for unique visitors, 181,892 and forty times the amount for visitor sessions, 230,446.

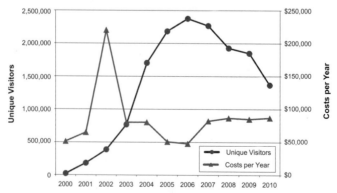

Fig. 4. Year end usage and costs for TeenHealthFX, considering 1999 through 2009.

In 2000, TeenHealthFX received a monthly average of 40 questions. In 2005, the monthly average was 567 and in 2009, 243 questions were received, on average, per month. **Fig. 5** shows the percentage of questions received by topic.

Considering 2008 traffic information, approximately 9% of users entered Teen-HealthFX by typing the URL address into an Internet browser, whereas 84% came to the Web site through an Internet search engine (eg, Google or Yahoo). The remaining 7% entered via a link from another Web site. Average visitors of TeenHealthFX spend just over 1 minute on the Web site and visit approximately 3 pages.

The most popular section of TeenHealthFX is the question-and-answer page of Sexuality & Sexual Health. In 2009, this section received more than 1.4 million page views and the 3 most popular questions clicked on in this category were "Vagina Hurts After Sex," "Penis Size," and "Pop The Cherry." Users spent an average of 1.5 minutes (94 seconds) on each of these pages. TeenHealthFX's sexuality category has 29 subsections and includes answers to more than 1400 questions. A common theme is, "Am I normal?" or "Is the activity that I am doing normal?" **Box 1** offers some examples of posted sexuality questions. The most frequently viewed questions concern masturbation and penis size.

Another popular TeenHealthFX section, receiving on average 3100 unique visitors per month in 2009, is the Advice from Teens page. This section is an area completely developed by adolescents who work on the TeenHealthFX TAC.

CONCERNS AND CONTROVERSY

When launching an adolescent health Web site, developers need to be cognizant of concerns and controversies already faced by others. Institutional lawyers and advisory boards raise issues around difficult, albeit infrequent, and highly sensitive issues, some of which need to be dealt with on an emergency basis. Often this is enough to dissuade Web site development. When the concept of TeenHealthFX was first raised, Atlantic Health System's lawyers and safety and security professionals were consulted. A primary concern was whether TeenHealthFX would be considered a crisis

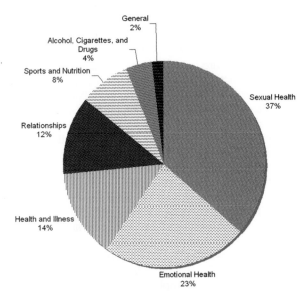

Fig. 5. Posted questions, by health topic, over the past 10 years of TeenHealthFX.

Box 1	
Examples of posted sex and sexuality questions	
11/19/2003	My girlfriend and I have started to have sex, and we use a condom. We're still a little nervous about her getting pregnant though, and she wants to be put on birth control, but she's afraid of getting examined. I was wondering if you could tell me what the examination for birth control consists of, and what I can do to help her through it.
5/23/2001	My boyfriend told me about a study that women who ingest semen have a lower risk of breast cancer. I have never heard this. Has there ever been that type of study done?
4/30/2002	When you measure your penis, Where do you start from? Do you take the ruler and start from the stomach and then measure out?
9/26/2002	I am a 16-year-old male. I have been masturbating since I was 15, and now excessive. Due to this my weight reduced and I have become very thin. My hair is also losing very fast. I really want to improve myself, by not doing this dirty act. I want to concentrate on studies as I am in 12th grade. Please help me.
2/5/2002	I am a 14-year-old girl. I have had my period since age 10. Since I was about 8 years I noticed that my nipples are significantly larger than my actual cup size. I wanted to know if this is normal, and if it will fill out, and if my breast cup will stay small or grow larger. Also I sometimes experience sharp pains that do not last long at all in all parts of my body, mostly my breasts. Does this mean that they are growing?

intervention Web site, and overt strategies were implemented to prevent this perception. Daily, round-the-clock monitoring was never intended nor is possible given financial and staffing constraints. As a result, policy and procedures were developed to address urgent matters, especially around threats to self and threats to others.

The top of TeenHealthFX's home page features a tab labeled "Emergency Help!" Clicking this tab brings users to a page with 3 telephone numbers displayed prominently, including (1) a 24-hour crisis hotline (for those living in Northern New Jersey), (2) 911 (for those outside Northern New Jersey), and (3) a toll-free suicide hotline. The toll-free number is the National Hopeline Network, and it connects to a local crisis hotline.

Web site staff, all of whom are trained pediatric health educators or mental health professionals, screen submitted questions daily (Monday through Friday). They flag suicide or violence-related remarks and adhere to the following protocol. First, a judgment is made as to the remark's seriousness and intent. Criteria, such as description of a specific plan, time frame, and location, are considered in this evaluation. Since its inception, TeenHealthFX has answered more than 141 questions dealing with suicide alone. It has answered 191 others on related topics, such as depression and cutting.

Staff also flag comments about abuse, homicide, or other threats, bringing these to the immediate attention of the director of security for the Atlantic Health System and the Web site's medical director, who is an adolescent medicine physician. With specific and credible threats, the hospital's local police department is notified. The police then decide whether to investigate further. Local authorities and law enforcement agencies then work with the Internet service provider host companies to identify the user's location. At this point, TeenHealthFX is no longer involved. Since the Web site has been live, TeenHealthFX and the Atlantic Health System have reported 16 comments to the police. As an example, the following remark, entitled "Lost All Interest in Life," was reported to authorities. It read,

This is probably pointless to ask but ill ask anyways, ive been a loner my whole life and ive been a target for other kids. ive never had a true friend and i have no idea what happiness is. I'm constantly confused and have anxiety attacks and i can hardly breathe because im now scared of everybody, afraid they will say something bad to me. my parents are no help either, they seem to hate me and say im an idiot and im good for nothing. im so miserable and ive been contemplating suicide for over 4 years now. i have nothing to live for and ive lost all interest in life; but now since ive been destroyed by others at school I feel like i want to kill them all. i understand why those kids did it at columbine, you can only take so much and your gonna snap. my problem is that, i cant get any help from anyone because im terrified, my life is so useless and if i don't do something soon, i think some people might wind up dead. what the hell am i supposed to do??

This comment was brought to attention of the hospital team and local law enforcement agencies, which took over the case.

TeenHealthFX faces two persistent, prominent, and controversial topics: marijuana use and abstinence-only sex education. Regarding marijuana use, the TeenHealthFX staff recognizes that use of this drug, although illegal, is common among adolescents. Answers posted on the Web site are factual and objective but also emphasize that relevant information exists describing that the potential harm associated with marijuana use. Counter to abstinence-only information and policies advanced by the US government during the past 10 years, TeenHealthFX advises that adolescents consider all their options. Although abstinence is suggested as a legitimate and healthy option, TeenHealthFX offers information on all contraceptive methods, sexually transmitted infections, and prevention of sexually transmitted infections.

Before the Web site's launch and at regular review times, philosophic and practical discussions occur among the TeenHealthFX team, including the Web site staff, medical director, hospital risk management, hospital attorney, director of safety and security, and law enforcement personnel. Noting the Web site's value, especially for troubled adolescents, there is an insistence to "do no harm." A high level of vigilance remains constant in monitoring the Web site, identifying situations of moral, ethical, and legal considerations.

THE EFFECT ON THE DEVELOPERS

The developers and maintainers of TeenHealthFX have experienced an additional positive effect. The Web site has enabled the professionals involved to have a clearer, more well informed sense of the concerns and thought processes of adolescents who use this health information resource. Through this venue, visitors express thoughts and submit questions that may not arise, even in the safest and most supportive in-person situations. Insights gained into adolescent thinking and behavior have the potential to improve the clinical interactions of the doctors, health educators, psychologists, and others involved with real-life youth.

TEENHEALTHFX AND THE FUTURE

Like similar Web sites, several challenges exist to the Web site's long-term prospects. First is ongoing funding and support. As discussed previously, this Web site was initially sponsored by the institution's Community Health Committee. Later, funding was rolled into the hospital system's operating budget. Monies through outside foundations or philanthropy have not been viable to date. The TeenHealthFX team, although regularly approached, has resisted commercial funding. It is believed that allowing companies, such as pharmaceutical or media companies, to reach youth through this Web site could taint the credibility and authenticity of the health material presented. It remains to be seen whether or not there may be a way to accept funding from outside sources while maintaining the Web site's integrity.

Another challenge facing TeenHealthFX is the evolving nature of technology. In the past decade, cell phones with extensive online features have emerged and become popular among adolescents. Ownership of cell phones among those 12 to 17 years old increased from one-third in 2003 to two-thirds in 2007.[11] Myspace and Facebook, two popular social networking Web sites, debuted in 2003 and 2004, respectively. In 2010, TeenHealthFX began using Twitter and Facebook with relevant posts daily. To stay current in 2012, TeenHealthFX will add a mobile application and alter its format so it is accessible via handheld devices.

SUMMARY

Over the past few decades (and perhaps over the past millennium), it has become clear that adolescents and technology are a good fit. Notwithstanding the real and perceived negative aspects of such media use, this case study is an example of how a Web site can be a valuable tool for young people. In addition to providing an accessible, anonymous, and nonpunitive resource for adolescents, TeenHealthFX has provided new insights regarding adolescent thinking and behavior for the professionals involved.

Many factors contributed to the success of this Web site and should be taken into account by anyone considering development of a similar project. TeenHealthFX began with a multidisciplinary team, including advisors from the local community and the target audience. This team provided an important foundation and set the stage for having persistent support and relevant advice. Although the costs involved have been substantial, the not-for-profit hospital system sponsoring the Web site has reaped direct and indirect benefits from providing this community service. Whether the costs will be worth it in the future is debatable. Technology is always evolving and the stark decreases in use might be a result in changing media activities among youth. In its next decade, TeenHealthFX will have to find new and innovative ways to deliver health information if it is going to continue benefiting its users and developers.

REFERENCES

1. Pew Internet, American Life Project. Generations online in 2009. Available at: http://www.pewinternet.org/Reports/2009/Generations-Online-in-2009.aspx. Accessed March 30, 2009.
2. Atkinson NL, Saperstein SL, Pleis J. Using the Internet for health-related activities: findings from a national probability sample. J Med Internet Res 2009;11(1):e4.
3. Borzekowski DL, Fobil JN, Asante KO. Online access by adolescents in Accra: Ghanaian teens' use of the Internet for health information. Dev Psychol 2006; 42(3):450–8.
4. Borzekowski DL, Rickert VI. Adolescent cybersurfing for health information: a new resource that crosses barriers. Arch Pediatr Adolesc Med 2001;155:813–7.
5. Tang PC, Lee TH. Your doctor's office or the Internet? Two paths to personal health records. N Engl J Med 2009;360:1276–8.
6. Eysenbach G, Englesakis M, Stern A. Health related virtual communities and electronic support groups: systematic review of the effects of online peer to peer interactions. Brit Med J 2004;328:1166–71.

7. Arunachalam S. Assuring quality and relevance of Internet information in the real world. Brit Med J 1998;317:1501–2.
8. Borzekowski DL, Rickert VI. Adolescents, the Internet, and health: issues of access and content. J Appl Dev Psych 2001;22:49–59.
9. Kanuga M, Rosenfeld WD. Adolescent sexuality and the internet: the good, the bad, and the URL. J Pediatr Adolesc Gynecol 2004;17:117–24.
10. Ginsburg KR, Menapace AS, Slap GB. Factors affecting the decision to seek health care: the voice of adolescents. Pediatrics 1997;100:922–30.
11. Experian Simmons. Teen tech use shapes consumer behavior. Available at: http://www.marketingcharts.com/interactive/teen-tech-use-shapes-consumer-behavior-7638/. Accessed November 24, 2009.

Index

Note: Page numbers of article titles are in **boldface** type.

Pediatr Clin N Am 59 (2012) 729–738
doi:10.1016/S0031-3955(12)00052-1
0031-3955/12/$ – see front matter © 2012 Elsevier Inc. All rights reserved.

pediatric.theclinics.com

Moving?

Make sure your subscription moves with you!

To notify us of your new address, find your **Clinics Account Number** (located on your mailing label above your name), and contact customer service at:

Email: journalscustomerservice-usa@elsevier.com

800-654-2452 (subscribers in the U.S. & Canada)
314-447-8871 (subscribers outside of the U.S. & Canada)

Fax number: 314-447-8029

Elsevier Health Sciences Division
Subscription Customer Service
3251 Riverport Lane
Maryland Heights, MO 63043

*To ensure uninterrupted delivery of your subscription, please notify us at least 4 weeks in advance of move.

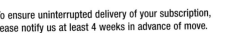
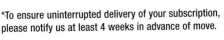